VENUS®

Summer

SHAPE UP

60 Days to Your Best Swimsuit Body

NOTICE

The *Venus Summer Shape Up* Program is intended as a reference volume provided for informational and educational purposes only. It is not a medical manual and is not intended to offer medical advice nor is it intended as a substitute for any treatment that may have been prescribed by your doctor. The food plan and exercise program are intended for healthy adults, age 18 and over. Before beginning this or any diet and exercise plan you should consult with your physician or health care provider. If you suspect you have a medical problem we urge you to seek help from competent medical personnel.

Mention of specific products or companies within this book does not imply endorsement by the author or publisher, nor that they in any way endorse the book, this program, the authors or the publisher.

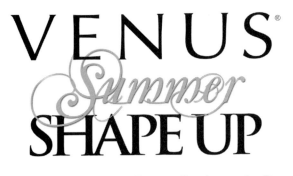

VENUS® Summer SHAPE UP

60 Days to Your Best Swimsuit Body

by

Daryle V. Scott, President of Venus Swimwear

Robert G. de Padua, M.D., Medical Consultant

Skip Sylvester, Personal Trainer and Bodybuilding Champion

I'd like to extend a heartfelt "Thank You" to those who worked so tirelessly to get this book completed on time. In particular, I'm grateful to Deborah Callaway for being the creative force behind the project, Brett Clark for his pre-press expertise, Vicki Floyd and Lynn Gerlach for their copy editing and proof reading assistance and most importantly to my very dear friend of 35 years, Carol Svec for lending her expertise, significant editing and constant counsel through-out the entire process.

I also want to extend my sincere gratitude to all of the dedicated employees of Venus for making my work life so fulfilling over so many years. You are indeed the best employees in the world.

About the Authors

Daryle Vlic Scott is Chief Executive Officer and President of Venus Swimwear (Venus.com). He has been professionally active in fitness since the early 1980s when he and four friends founded Titan Bodybuilding, a company that evolved into Venus Swimwear in 1984. Fitness has always been a passion of Daryle's, and he was a competitive power lifter from 1986 to 1991, but readily admits that he was only average at best. During his tenure as President and CEO of Venus, Daryle has worked with and interviewed literally hundreds of swimwear models and he knows the secrets they use to stay in shape.

Daryle's exercise routine includes lifting weights 3 to 4 days per week (one hour per session), biking 8 to 10 miles 5 nights per week, and playing tennis twice each week. Daryle is also an avid snow skier and skis in Colorado as much as his busy schedule allows.

Skip Sylvester has been the fitness coordinator for Venus Swimwear for the past 13 years. In 1983, he began power lifting and bodybuilding. He has won numerous titles, including Southern States Power Lifting Champion, Mr. Northeast Florida Bodybuilding Champion, Central Florida Bench Press Champion, and All Star Classic of Florida Over 40 Champion. In 2003, the North Florida Bodybuilding Association presented Skip with a Lifetime Achievement Award. Currently, Skip owns and runs a personal training business, Body by Skip, Inc. (bodybyskipinc.com). His client base is several hundred strong and includes professional athletes, celebrities, and dignitaries.

Skip's workout program consists of weight training 3 days per week, alternating between a power building and a circuit training routine. His cardiovascular routine is a combination of low-impact and interval training 5 times per week.

Robert G. de Padua, M.D., is a physician in private practice specializing in Internal Medicine. He is the medical consultant for Venus Swimwear, and also for Brumos Porsche Racing and Anheuser-Busch in Jacksonville, Florida. He was formerly a medical consultant for local branches of the F.B.I., Secret Service, and the U.S. Marshals.

Robert works out 3 times per week with 20 to 30 minutes of cardio training consisting of calisthenics and running stairs, and 20 to 30 minutes of light weightlifting.

Table of Contents

The *Venus* Philosophy

At *Venus*, everyday is bikini day.

Depending on how you feel about your body, putting on a bikini can be either thrilling or horrifying. The purpose of this book is to get you in the best shape of your life so you no longer feel the need to cover up your luscious curves. We want you to feel comfortable and confident about your body, just as our models do. We want you back on the beach!

The *Venus Summer Shape Up* is a custom-designed weight loss and fitness plan created by a team of experts that includes me, internal medicine specialist Dr. Bobby de Padua, certified personal trainer and bodybuilding champion Skip Sylvester, and the world's top experts in looking fabulous— our very own *Venus* models.

Why swimwear models, you ask? Simple. If you want to be a gourmet cook, take lessons from top chefs who cook gourmet meals for a living. If you want to be a top tennis player, take lessons from a pro. And if you want to improve your physique, you'll get the best advice from professional swimwear models, women who make their living with a slim, toned, well-maintained body.

By following our proven program, bolstered by model-approved tips and techniques that have been proven successful in season after season of *Venus* catalog shoots, you will have the tools to transform yourself, head to toe, inside and out. You'll be leaner, stronger, and healthier. You will be more confident. I guarantee it.

I'm going to share with you secrets and tips I've seen used by dozens of our models over the past 25 years, and, in special chapters throughout the book, you'll read profiles of three of my favorite models: Rocky, Rachel, and

Jessiqa. Through their personal stories, they inspire, educate, and provide living proof that having a sleek shape is possible no matter your age, how many children you've had, or what other personal obstacles you've faced. Their message is this:

Everyone can have a better bikini-body.
All it takes is passion, focus, and a little bit of sweat.

I know what you're thinking—you didn't count on having to sweat. A lot of people are making buckets of money selling weight-loss plans that require no work, no dieting, and no exercise. In a word: Impossible! But these people get away with it because they use the magic word, the one all of us secretly want to read every time we open a new weight loss book or watch the latest "miracle" infomercial: *Easy.* They claim that all you need is this new pill or new miracle supplement. But if all of those miracle solutions really worked, if it were really so "easy" to lose weight, why are we in the middle of an obesity epidemic?

The fact is that 99.9% of women (and men) are not born genetically gifted in the body department. Are you? Can you eat whatever you want, as much as you want, sit around all day and still manage to look lean and fit? No? Well, join the club. Not even swimwear models have that kind of freedom. But if they are going to stay in the profession, models don't have a choice— they must maintain a certain discipline in order to create that appearance of being effortlessly perfect. For a model, losing her physique would be the equivalent of a scientist losing her brain. They are paid for how they look, so they do the work required to look great. The good news for the rest of us is that what they do isn't magic and it isn't impossible. There are secrets and tips which we're going to share with you. Armed with that information and a little motivation, you can do it too.

The reality is that although the rest of us care about how we look, our livelihood doesn't depend on it. We try to shape up, but it's tough, especially if you have to conquer more than just your waistline. Many women have problems dealing with their own personal diet demons, such as:

• *Confusing skinniness with beauty.* "Skeletal Skinny" may be chic on high fashion runways, but not in the real world...and definitely not at *Venus*. Here, we value healthy beauty. Our models are attractive, in shape, and have a body mass index that is in the normal range. Personally, I don't understand the fashion designers who hang their beautiful creations on clothes hanger-sized anorexic women who look as if they eat no more than a single shrimp a day. Who wants to live like that? And more importantly, who really wants to look like that? No men I know find that look attractive, and the average woman isn't fooled. She wants to look beautiful, shapely, slender, and healthy, but not runway-model skinny. That's the goal of this program. We can help you get there, and we can show you results if you'll give us just 60 days.

• *Collecting diet books without committing to any of them.* I'll let you in on a secret: You can't absorb information by osmosis. I'm joking, of course, but you would be surprised by how many people—men and women alike—collect diet books the way some folks collect stamps. Each new volume gets stuck on a shelf with the books they bought last year, the year before, and the year before that. What happens is that we get excited to finally start a diet we think will work, but when we open the book, our motivation gets sapped before we even begin because the diet looks more complex than we bargained for, or

The Venus Summer Shape Up

there is too much blah-blah-blah reading to wade through before getting to the good stuff. We're going to fix those problems by giving you a single program with clear, illustrated steps and examples and no excess fluff to sift through. On every page, you'll find valuable information to keep you motivated and committed.

• *Shifting priorities.* Life is complicated. And busy. But every day we have the opportunity to choose our priorities and change our lives. If losing weight and becoming fit are important to you, put those activities at the top of your priority list...and keep them there! Look, I know you've heard this before but it bears repeating: We ALL have only 24 hours in a day. And today it seems as if life is busier than ever. A good friend of mine calls it "noise." We have things we want to do and we have things that we think should be a priority but the "noise" of life is distracting, and we find ourselves spending our 24 hours on things other than the ones we claim to be our top priorities. I've heard people say, "I just don't have time to work out." I ask those people how much TV they watch each day and they'll usually say, "ONLY an hour or two." Well, if you've got an hour or two to watch TV, you have plenty of time to do the work our models do—but only if you make doing that work—and having a beautiful swimwear body—a priority. Lack of time is never an acceptable excuse. Don't worry, we'll show you ways to avoid the temptation to let your goals slip down the list.

- *Looking for a permanent fix.* Like anything worthwhile, fitness requires dedication and attention. And once you attain your ultimate goal, you have to maintain it. Good health is not like climbing a mountain where you put in the effort early so you can rest at the top. Instead, it's more like keeping a clean house—it can be perfect one day, but if you want to keep it pristine, you have to continue to apply effort and keep on top of it. Once you get your ideal body, you need to keep up your new, healthy lifestyle. Later in the book, we'll tell you how to maintain your best body once all your hard work has paid off.

- *Thinking in the short-term.* A friend of mine started taking piano lessons as a teenager but abandoned them after about a year because it was too hard to find the time to practice. Although she had been making steady progress, the learning process was too slow for her. Now, as an adult, she looks back and realizes that if she had kept up the lessons during the ensuing 20 years, she'd be pretty darned talented by now. It's the same with diet programs. Too many people abandon their dreams of a better body because it feels too difficult at the moment. But time will pass, and what you do today makes a big difference tomorrow. Think of it this way: What do you want for your life? Do you want to stay in the same shape you are in now (or worse!), or do you want to be fit and gorgeous? Whatever you want tomorrow (or this summer) you have to start working on today, and we can put you on the right path and show you a REAL difference in just 60 days!

Are you ready to be strong and bold and confident?

Are you ready to transform your body and your life?

The *Venus Summer Shape Up* can help you bust through all these barriers. The program offers *quick results,* and if you commit to doing the work, *you will have a different, better body in 60 days.* You won't starve, and it is entirely possible that *you could drop two sizes or more in just 60 days.* Let our models inspire and motivate you to make this the one diet book you keep on the coffee table; not on the shelf.

Dayle V. Scott

Section One ———

Preparation

Chapter 1:
Attitude is Half the Battle

What is your secret (or not-so-secret) passion?

Everybody has one. What is the thing that sparks your interest and gives you energy even when you're bone-tired; that defines who you are because it lives at the very core of your self? Is it family, or maybe your work, or reading, gardening, cleaning, swimming, tanning, or shopping? Think about it for a moment.

Now, close your eyes and try to remember a time when you were fully engaged in your passion, doing what you love. Try to remember how you felt while you were having that perfect moment. Got it? How many of these feelings did you experience?

- ✓ Happy
- ✓ Calm
- ✓ Energetic
- ✓ Powerful
- ✓ Free
- ✓ Excited
- ✓ Satisfied
- ✓ Inspired
- ✓ Confident

Having a passion makes life more vivid—sort of like that point in the *Wizard of Oz* when Dorothy leaves black-and-white Kansas and lands in an exciting, Technicolor® world. Everything appears brighter, and you *feel* different and better!

Now here's the good news:

It is possible to create a passion for fitness.

It's true! In fact, you can create a passion for just about anything, so you might as well use that ability to become passionate about working on positive change for your body. In its simplest form, passion requires a combination of clear focus, active pursuit, and both short-term and long-term goals. In other words:

Focus + Pursuit + Goals = Passion

Let's break it down…

Focus

If you look hard enough, you can find something to enjoy in just about anything. You may have to get out a high-powered microscope to locate it, but it's there.

Take exercise, for example. Instead of concentrating on how much you don't want to get up off the couch, make a mental **shift**—focus instead on some tiny thing you like about working out. It doesn't even have to be about the activity itself. Why do you think so many women buy new outfits when they begin a new fitness program? Their point of focus starts with the clothing, and there's nothing wrong with that. Some women buy colorful, vinyl-coated hand weights because they are not only more comfortable, but cute, too. Others love having a chance to leave their desks and walk

18

outside…or the feeling of power that comes from moving up to a higher-weight dumbbell…or the natural exhilaration that comes from aerobic exercise…or meeting friends to work out together…or having the time to listen to all the tracks on their iPods. You get the picture.

Find a focus that works for you. That's your **"spark."** Concentrate on it; zoom in like a laser. That one spark—no matter how small—can ignite real passion, but you have to add the next part of the equation: Pursuit.

Pursuit

Once you find your spark, you have to take action. If you leave a spark alone too long, it fizzles out. To keep it alive, you need to engage it, work with it and allow it to become part of you. Passion doesn't always come naturally or automatically, so you have to pursue it. Start by chasing your spark. If your spark is a new outfit, don't just go out and buy track shoes only to let them gather dust in the closet—use them! Every time you put those shoes on to exercise, you fan the spark so it can grow to become a full-blown passion.

Of course, empty activity won't get you very far without goals.

Goals

The final variable in the passion equation consists of the short-term and long-term goals you set for yourself. Every choice you make today affects what happens to you tomorrow, next year, and ten years from now. Small choices, actions that may seem insignificant now, will have an impact that changes the entire course of your life. Imagine a tree....

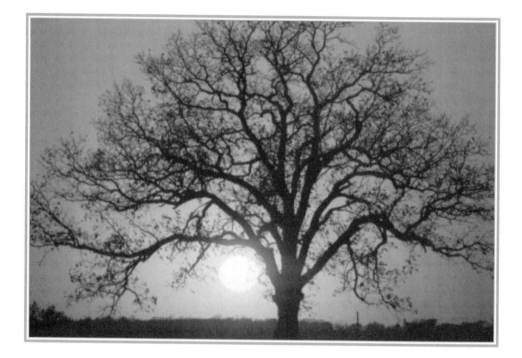

Notice that there are thousands of branches, and those branches have branches, and the branches on those branches have branches. Our lives are like that tree. As you climb, you make choices about which branch to walk out on. Sometimes you can change your mind and walk back, but often the decisions are irreversible, and you can only move on from where you are. Eventually, your journey stops at the tip of a twig on a branch on a limb of your own personal life tree. And that, my friend, is your life.

Where you end up is almost purely a consequence of the decisions you make along the way. Sure, some events are beyond your control, but even then, there is almost always another branch to climb. So the question you need to start with is this:

Where do I want to end up?

Choose an end point on the illustrated tree. Maybe it's a place you think looks the most interesting, or offers the best view, or allows you to climb farther than you ever thought you could. Starting at the tip of the twig that is your end point, trace a path back to the trunk. Notice that there is only one possible route; a single path from branch to branch that gets you to where you want to be. Now, take a moment to examine all the other possible branches that lead away from your chosen goal. The point is that we make many life choices, but if we want to reach our ultimate goal, we have to keep moving in the direction that offers us the best chance of getting there. That's your *tree path*.

Now, let's translate all of that to the real world, and to health in particular.

What do you want for your body?

If you want to lose weight, become fit, improve your strength and energy, and finally feel comfortable in a swimsuit, then that's your goal. Remember it, and do what you need to do to get there. So many times we become sidetracked by the pull of a short-term desire, such as wanting a cheeseburger or a bowl of ice cream. But eating a cheeseburger or ice cream won't take you to your goal of wearing a bikini, will it? It's not that different from the person who is trying to quit smoking, but buys a pack of cigarettes "just in case." In case of what? In case she decides her future isn't worth it? Yes, a cheeseburger tastes good going down, and you're going to feel good for the five minutes it takes to eat it, but that choice is only going to derail your climb to your goal. (Don't worry – we'll give you a chance to have the occasional cheeseburger or bowl of ice cream! You don't have to give up ANYTHING forever on our program. You just can't indulge every day.)

When it comes to fitness, we all have to develop longer-term vision. See the outcome you want in your mind, and then choose to take that one path that gets you there. It may be very different from the path you are on now, but change is what you are really looking for. There's a great saying I recall from one of my college psychology classes: "You can't do what you've always done and not expect to get what you've always got." Translated: *If you want a different outcome; if you want a different physique, you MUST make different decisions.*

Look in the mirror. The decisions you've made in the past have led you to where you are today. And if you're reading this book, odds are that you want to change something about that person in the mirror. That means you need to start making different decisions.

It Starts with Attitude

None of this can happen if you don't approach the process with a good attitude.

When people talk about attitude, they mean the particular state of mind you bring to a situation. A person with a "good attitude" is positive, open-minded, enthusiastic, and willing to try anything that will allow her to reach her goals. It is a state of readiness that makes a passionate pursuit of a goal possible. Remember:

Passion = Focus + Pursuit + Goals

When you focus on your spark of enjoyment—become active in pursuing the passion while keeping your ultimate goal and "tree path" in mind—you create a small fire of passion. But a bad attitude distorts all of it. If you believe nothing good will ever happen…that diets don't work for you…that you'll never wear a bikini…then, guess what? You're right. A bad attitude is a passion killer. It smothers any spark that ignites. And if you don't develop a spark and a passion for exercise and eating right, you're not going to stick with it for very long—kind of like that boyfriend or husband you dropped because the passion faded. You can pretend for awhile, but eventually you just move on.

The rest of this book gives you specific information about The *Venus Summer Shape Up*. **It works.** It can help you get the body you want. You'll glow with vibrant good health. Remember the secrets to success:

Begin with a desire
Adjust your attitude
Find that spark
Remember your tree path
Develop a passion for fitness

Start creating the body you've always wanted!

Chapter 2:
From Wake-Up Call to the Beach

Because this diet program was inspired by models, it made sense to recreate a day in the life of a model at a photo shoot. Here's how you can follow in their footsteps:

While on location for a *Venus* photo shoot, a model's day starts with a **wake-up call**—often as early as 3:30 am! That's because the light is softer and more flattering first thing in the morning when the sun has just come up, so the models need to be ready in time to catch those gentle rays. No excuses, no lounging around—the models have to drag themselves out of bed well before dawn to start work. (Still think models have a cushy life?)

Next, the model undergoes a **transformation.** With the help of hair stylists and make-up artists, the model's facial look is perfected. It's too late to fix the body; the model either has it or she doesn't! Finally, she puts on a swimsuit from the new design season, applies body lotion, and she's ready to be photographed.

As she heads to the location, our model prepares for the photo shoot by becoming mentally and physically **energized.** She has spent most of the morning getting ready for this moment. She knows that to look her best—to make our apparel looks its best—she needs to focus, pay attention to every detail of her look, and project her personality to the lens. Beauty really does start on the inside. The camera can tell if a model is "on" and "up". No matter how she really may feel, she has to act "up" and "energized." And guess what? If you want to feel a certain way you can start by acting as if you feel that way and pretty soon you may find you're not acting! You really do feel that way. Fake it 'til you make it!

By the time the model arrives at **The Beach,** she looks gorgeous and is ready to do what she does best—make our *Venus* swimwear look sexy and fabulous.

The *Venus Summer Shape Up* is divided into three phases named after a typical model's day:

Phase 1—Wake-up Call

Phase 2—Transformation

Phase 3—Energizing

Ultimately, the goal is to get to "The Beach." For models, that means being in top bikini shape for a photo shoot. What does it mean for you?

Defining Your Personal "Beach"

We all use goals to inspire and guide us. A goal can influence your decisions, your motivation, and the course of your life.

For example, if your goal is to become a doctor, you have to take science classes in college, get good grades, apply and go to medical school, then complete an internship and residency. The process requires focus, dedication, and a lot of hard work. It guides everything you do for years. Years! And yet, the fulfillment of that dream—reaching that particular branch on your life tree—is worth the effort.

Because you are reading this book, you obviously have a general goal to lose weight or improve your fitness. Let's make that more specific: How much weight do you want to lose? Is there a special event you are shaping up for? What is your ideal, ultimate goal?

**Whatever you want, whatever you dream of,
that is your Beach, your destination.
That is what you are working for.**

A lot of diet books will tell you that it's a bad idea to focus on losing weight for a special event, that you need to think long-term, yadda yadda. Really? Think about it—having a specific goal can motivate you to try harder. As long as the goal is important to you, having something real and measurable to reach for will carry you through those times when you might feel like giving up.

Model Secret!

Even if models don't have a shoot date booked, they will pretend that they have one and work toward that date just as if it were a real booking. So if you don't have any particular event coming up you can either create an event or pretend (like our models do) that some event is coming up. Plan or pretend you have a swimsuit party coming up. Plan to attend your next high school reunion. Or set a date to have your photo taken by a professional photographer. If it serves as motivation for you, then use it!

Years ago, I competed in power lifting contests. Although I had worked out hard for years and years, I never worked harder than when I knew I had a contest coming up in six months. That contest—that important event—served as motivation for me to put in extra effort to achieve my goal. For our models, the goal may be the next photo shoot. For you, it may be an upcoming pool party, a class reunion, or just a desire to go to the beach this summer and hear the admiring compliments from your friends. Specific events and solid goals can help keep you focused.

Having a goal is like having a job. We all have something that motivates us to keep getting up and going to work everyday—maybe it's family, maybe it's the rent we have to pay, maybe it's that new pair of Christian Louboutin pumps. Or maybe it's the satisfaction of doing well at a job we love, or spending time with coworkers who are also friends. But there is always something…nobody works for nothing. The lesson is this:

In order to have the best chance of success, you must define your goal.

What is your weight loss or fitness goal? Be as specific as possible. Do you want to lose 10 pounds? Get in shape before a cruise? Fit into that cute dress you saw at the mall? Or maybe you want to look like Jessica Alba, Denise Austin, Carmen Electra, Scarlett Johansson, or one of the *Venus* models. Or maybe you just want to look more like you did when you were in high school.

What is your goal? Don't worry about how unrealistic it might seem right now, you need a place to start. Why not try for what you really want? Remember…

If you reach for the stars, you might not quite get one, but you won't end up with a handful of mud, either.
(Leo Burnett)

The lesson is that it is better to dream big and risk having only partial success than to settle for what you already have. Who do you want to see when you look in the mirror? What is your ultimate weight loss or fitness goal, your "Beach"? Write it down here:

_____

Now let's get you there. Let's get you to the Beach! Have you ever heard the phrase, "A goal without a plan is just a dream"? Knowing where you want to go is not enough, you also need good directions. That's what this book is about.

Your goal philosophy

Time for a short quiz. For each statement, choose the answer that most closely matches your experience or opinion.

1. If I have a big project to complete in a week, I like to:

   a. Decide in advance how much I want to get done each day so I know I'll make the deadline.

   b. Jump in and start the work without worrying about day-to-day progress.

2. My ability to focus is strongest:

   a. When I have a clear view of the goal, and it seems easily attainable.

   b. When I have a clear view of the goal, no matter how difficult it seems.

3. When I read a book:

   a. I almost always break at the end of a chapter.

   b. I stop when I stop, even if it is in the middle of a chapter.

If you chose answer (a) to complete two or three of the statements, then you are the kind of person who finds success by using short-term goals to mark your progress on your way to an ultimate goal.

If you chose answer (b) to complete two or three of the statements, then you are the kind of person who drives straight to the ultimate goal, without concern for intermediate goals.

Enjoying the short-term rewards

Imagine that you are driving from Florida to California. It is natural to look for signposts — markers that show where you are and that you are making progress. As you drive through Texas and reach the New Mexico border, you know that you are one state closer to your destination, and it's a cause for celebration. I know some people who honk the horn as they cross a state border, and others who make a game of seeing who can enter the state "first" by reaching their hands forward when they pass the Welcome sign.

People who enjoy using short-term rewards on their way to their destination look for these kinds of checkpoints because they are helpful. If this is you, then short-term goals are the rungs on your ladder; the individual steps you need to take to get where you want to go. These mini-goals make the larger, more difficult goals seem manageable. Plus, there's the added bonus of more frequent victory celebrations!

Feel free to use short-term goals if they are helpful to you. Set goals as small as you need, as often as you need. It is important to understand your personal philosophy and the way you work best, and then find a strategy that works best for you. It could mean the difference between losing the weight you want or giving up too early. For example, the other day a girl in the gym was complaining that she had watched her diet and worked out hard all week, but she lost ONLY 3 pounds. She felt like that was a disaster, and that she had somehow failed. But what if she could lose the same amount of weight every week for the next 3 months? Twelve weeks, at 3 pounds per week is a loss of almost 40 pounds. That's huge! Losing those 3 pounds was the first step to success, but in her mind it was a failure because she wanted massive and immediate results. She had been hoping to lose at least 10 pounds. Maybe some people can lose that in a week, but that much weight loss is mostly water weight, and not a loss of 10 pounds of "fat." But 3 pounds per week is a solid result that should make anyone proud.

Whether you like to use short-term goals or go immediately for the whole enchilada, keep your personal goals at the forefront of your mind. Make them so real that you can visualize them when you close your eyes. If it helps to cut a picture out of a magazine or to locate a picture of YOU when you were in great shape to inspire you, do it. Tape it to your refrigerator! But only if that kind of motivation helps you—some people find it more frustrating than helpful. This is your opportunity to decide who you want to be tomorrow. And then you have to get moving! No one is going to pick you up in a helicopter and bring you to the Beach. You have to get there yourself, under your own power.

A note about the "quick fix"

Yes, we know there are ads and commercials and infomercials offering miracle weight-loss solutions. They promise that you can "take a magic pill and watch the pounds melt off," or "listen to our secret and you'll be able to simply wish your thighs away." Well, we say, "Bull!" The only thing all those miracle solutions really do is make a lot of money for the manufacturer or promoter. They take advantage of the natural desire for easy answers. Sorry folks, there are no miracles in achieving weight loss and fitness. There are no easy answers. Our models get paid well to be in shape. If there were an easy, no-sweat, no-effort way to get in shape, they would know what it was, and they would use it. But there isn't. Weight loss is totally possible, but it will take all of the elements working together—focus, goals, and the active pursuit of a dream. If that sounds a little…well…scary, please don't worry—we have the plan.

The *Venus Summer Shape Up*

Our program has a diet component and an exercise component. These two pieces of the fitness puzzle make a complete picture. Studies have shown that diet alone works for a limited time, for reasons you'll read about in chapter 4. Exercise alone can make you fit and strong, but exercise by itself doesn't help you lose much weight. But if you put diet and exercise together, the results are explosive—a new body...*in as little as 60 days.*

Our program is divided into three phases that build upon each other. Each phase lasts 20 days, so in less than 3 weeks, you move one step closer to your goal. To help everyone succeed, the program defines which foods are healthy and which foods are off-limits. And because you'll be eating 5 times a day, you'll never be hungry.

PHASE 1: Wake-Up Call

Everybody needs a wake-up call once in a while. This first phase of the program is designed to regulate your appetite and break bad habits. It also will ease you into a body-shaping exercise program.

PHASE 2: Transformation

By the time you reach this phase, your body will already be different. Even your taste buds will have changed. Foods you used to crave before you started the program won't interest you quite as much. In this phase, some of the dietary restrictions are lifted, and you step up to the next intensity level in your work-out.

PHASE 3: Energizing

In this final phase, you will discover a new state of happiness. When was the last time you actually *liked* your body? In this phase, you will have already begun to transform into the person you always wanted to be. As you become stronger, firmer, and slimmer, you'll find that you've changed more than just your waist and thighs—your outlook on life will have also changed. You're one step closer to the Beach.

Final Note

You may be tempted to skip Sections One and Two and jump right to Section Three with the plan details. Unless you have been working out regularly, we don't recommend that. Information is so important in understanding program specifics. If you are already a work-out fanatic and eat relatively healthfully, feel free to skip ahead...but please come back and read the information about metabolism, eating, aerobic exercise, and resistance training. When you understand how the puzzle pieces fit together, you are more likely to stick with the program. You'll be less likely to skip exercise days or "cheat" on the diet (other than during your allowed "Free Day"). And don't miss our three model stories on pages 33, 66, and 183. These women are an inspiration, and have tips that can help you reach *your* Beach.

Chapter 3:
A Model Story—Rocky

> Rocky was one of the first *Venus* models, and she epitomizes our philosophy of *health first*. Because Rocky packs a big personality in her tiny frame, she leaves a lasting impression on everyone who works with her.

I always wanted to model. My first job was at age 10 when I modeled in one of those mall fashion shows. From the minute I stepped on a runway, I knew I had found my true calling, and I wasn't going to let anything stand in my way. I did a bunch of ads for JC Penney's, Sears, and Gold Circle department stores—remember Gold Circle? As I grew older, it became clear that I was going to be "vertically challenged." I started small and stayed small. I topped out at 5'3", when most models range between 5'8" and 5'11". But I didn't let my height bother me at all—I was determined to be a model.

When I was 18, my sister entered me in a *Venus* Swimwear Pageant. I was living in Chicago at the time, and I had done some local swimsuit modeling, but nothing big, so I wasn't convinced that bikinis were in my future. One day, I visited my family back in Ohio, and my sister took me to a club. Once we were inside, she pulled a swimsuit out of her handbag and all but pushed me on stage for a modeling contest. Imagine my surprise when I won, and received a free trip to Florida to participate in the finals. My parents flew down to cheer me on and generally make a big deal about it. For me, it was about the biggest thing in my life!

I ended up not winning…not a runner-up…not even in the top 10. I placed somewhere in the top 20. But the owner of the company and the photographer saw something in me. I think they could see my desire, and they gave me my first big job modeling swimwear for a *Venus* catalog. I still remember getting on the plane to go to Jamaica for the photo shoot. I had never been out of the country before. Even now, it gives me goose bumps just thinking about it—it was so surreal to go from Chicago to that exotic tropical beach. (The other model on this adventure, Wendy, became one of my absolute best friends!) The whole experience was better than anything I could have dreamed.

I worked for *Venus* as a swimwear model for 9 years—that's a long time in this business. During that time, I also worked as an actress. I appeared in many TV series, including *Silk Stalkings, Wings, Port Charles, Renegade,* and *Beyond Belief,* and quite a few movies, including *Species II, Fever, Mother Ghost,* and *A Night at the Roxbury.*

My beauty philosophy

It goes to show, it doesn't matter if you don't fit the mold…it doesn't matter if people tell you to give up. What matters is that you believe in yourself, do the work, and actively chase your dream. And it doesn't matter if you win or lose, it's what you do with the opportunities you are given. I may be a good six inches shorter than most models, but I've found a way to make my vision real.

Although you might not guess it by looking at my pictures, I've always had to work hard to maintain my body. What can I say—I'm Italian, and I like food. Bread, especially. And dark chocolate. And among my friends, I'm known as the Chocolate Chip Cookie Queen. The weight used to settle around my thighs, but in my 30s, it shifted. Now when I gain, it's more around my mid-section, and it is much, *much* harder to lose it. I've learned that I really can't ever let my weight get out of hand. No one gains 50 pounds overnight! It happens one pound at a time. For me, it is far easier to take care of the problem when I gain 5 pounds rather than wait until I've gained 25.

Model Secret!

Models never let themselves get too far out of shape before getting really serious about bringing their bodies back in line. Most models have a cutoff of 5 pounds. If they find they've gained 5 pounds, they get serious about their workouts and diet that day. They never wait until they've gained 10 pounds. Once you reach your goal, set your own 5-pound cutoff, and use the scale to help you decide when to get a little more strict with your diet and exercise.

To take care of myself, I (like most models) have to watch what I eat and work out regularly. I don't do it to be "skinny"…I do it because it feels good, and I've made it part of my life, starting from way back. I remember doing Jane Fonda routines back when I was 14!

My "tricks"

There are no real tricks to staying slim and healthy, but I do have a few personal habits that I think help.

Just as we were taught in school, I believe that breakfast is the most important meal of the day because it starts your metabolism. When you get up, your body is "starving" and your metabolism is at a crawl. You have to teach your body that you are not starving and give your body a reason to start up the metabolism engine. When I get up and have a nice breakfast, I have energy all day long, and it gets my metabolism started. I'll also have lunch and dinner, and I'll snack on little things between meals, but I don't gain weight because my metabolism is always working. That's the best.

Usually, I'll have a protein shake with fruit, or sometimes granola for my snacks. If I'm in a hurry, I might have a protein bar. But I always make time for breakfast. Not only does it get my metabolism started, but if I don't have time for breakfast, I crash. For example, yesterday was crazy. I had two auditions in the morning, so I had to run out of the house, then rush to see a friend to help him solve a crisis, and before I knew it, it was 4pm. I was so tired and felt really crappy. It's not good for me to do that to my body.

I've also noticed that when I eat smaller meals and eat slowly, I get full faster. And if I'm enjoying the company I'm with, I don't eat as much—I don't scarf the food down. When I sit down to a meal, I like to take it in, savor it. I think it's important to take the time to enjoy what you are doing at that moment. You'll notice you chew slower, eat slower, get fuller faster, and you won't gobble up everything on your plate. And you don't need to! Stop trying to eat everything on your plate! Parents used to preach about the "Clean Plate Club," but it's really a horrible habit, and it's not necessary. Whether you clean your plate or throw out the extras, the food that was on your plate can't help anyone starving anywhere else. By eating everything, you are not helping anyone and you're actually hurting yourself. Have courage and be willing to throw out the extra. This is especially important in restaurants, where a single plate can hold enough food to feed a family! Don't be fooled into trying to eat it all. You can reduce the temptation by asking the server to bring only half the meal to you on a plate, and immediately wrap the other half "to go" without ever putting that second half on your plate.

When I have to get ready for a modeling job, I cut out all breads and anything with refined white flour for three days before the shoot. That takes away a lot of foods I really like to eat, so I can't help but eat healthier by totally avoiding those foods that I KNOW are bad for me.

As for exercise, I do a lot of different things because I want to make it fun. Ideally, I try to work out for 1 hour a day, 5 times per week. If I need it (like after a rare cookie-fest), or if I have time on my hands, I'll do up to 2 hours per day. If I'm in a gym, I do 20 minutes of work on my abs, 45 minutes of cardio, and then spend the rest of the time on strength training. I also love doing Pilates—it's tough, but it lengthens and tones you, and builds your core muscles.

I like to change it up. If my mind is getting bored, then my body is getting bored, too. If your body is bored, your fitness will reach a plateau. If you do the same routine the same way every time, it is so monotonous…your body will get used to it and you won't see an improvement. But if you change it, you'll start feeling sore in places you never knew you had! When I started doing yoga, I couldn't move in the morning because I was so sore. I love that feeling because it means I'm really working my body.

In the summertime I do a lot of hiking outside—that's an amazing cardio-vascular workout, especially here in California where there are a lot of hills. It's really good on the thighs and butt. If you grab a few 2-pound hand-weights, you get an all-over workout.

Between modeling, acting, and being a spokesperson, I'm always traveling. If I pack a yoga DVD or Pilates DVD, I can get a good workout in any hotel room. Sometimes I bring resistance bands so I can tone muscles anywhere I am.

Where I am now

I think everything works together—philosophy, food, exercise. Being in shape has definite benefits now, but I'm also concerned with improving my longevity. My life is about more than just modeling. I'm always trying something new. Right now, I'm creating an animal show for kids. I'm writing and producing…I didn't know I had it in me! I'm also getting back into acting more. I just finished a film called *Rockett* with Jimmy Fallon, Sharon Stone, and Tom Arnold. Such cool people. I also have a really supportive family. My parents are my best friends—also cool people. Oh, and there's my constant buddy, my Persian cat, Zaide.

I believe it is important to have a strong faith and sense of spirit within myself. If you have something to believe in, it's easier to have a positive outlook on life and to keep your drive, regardless of any obstacles. I think it all plays a part in staying healthy. It's important to me to take care of my body. It's the only one I have…and I want to be around a long time.

Rocky's model secrets…

- Doesn't let obstacles stand in the way of her dreams.

- Belief in herself has allowed her to succeed.

- Has to work hard to maintain her body.

- Loves food—especially bread and chocolate—but doesn't eat to excess.

- Has never wanted to be skinny—she likes the fit look.

- Eats breakfast every day to start up her metabolism.

- Favorite "power snacks" are protein bars, protein shakes with fruit, or granola.

- Enjoys dining with friends.

- Doesn't believe in the "Clean Plate Club."

- Before a photo shoot, she abstains from eating sweets and carbs for 3 days.

- Works out 5 days per week, one hour per day (more if she over-indulges).

- Her workout includes 20 minutes of abdominal work and about 45 minutes of cardio. She also enjoys yoga and Pilates.

Section Two
Understanding

Chapter 4:
Head-First Eating

One of the most common questions asked of doctors and nutritionists alike is, "I want to lose weight—can you tell me what to eat?" It's kind of a funny question because most of the time, people really do know exactly what to eat and, more importantly, what NOT to eat! Here is proof in the form of a pop quiz. For each pair of foods, which is the healthier choice?

Cupcake or Apple?

Sausage pizza or Green salad?

Salami or Salmon?

Ice cream or Yogurt?

Blueberry muffin or Broccoli?

White bread or Whole wheat bread?

Cheeseburger or Grilled Chicken?

The correct answer for each of the pairs is the second option (of course). Chances are you already knew that, and no doubt found the quiz quite easy.

So we already know the basics. We know the difference between "healthy" and "unhealthy", "wrong" and "right," "good" and "bad" foods. If your friend asked, you could probably tell *her* what foods to eat and what foods to avoid if she wanted to lose weight, right? But knowing isn't the same as doing. You probably know someone (yourself, maybe?) who has made a vow to eat nothing but "good" foods from now on, or at least until they reached some goal weight, but managed to last only a day or two before cracking and eating a "bad" food—something that was so obviously unhealthy that there was no way it was a mistake. The diet breaks almost before it begins. And often, once you make that first "mistake," you immediately give up and think of yourself as a failure. We solve this by allowing you to "make a mistake" at prescribed times.

When people decide to go on a diet, what they really want is a plan that works fast so they can lose a ton of weight, and then they want to go back to eating the way they did before. Unfortunately, the usual diet for many of us emphasizes all things sugary, doughy, greasy, fatty, saucy, salty, and chocolate. That kind of "eat-what-you-want" diet doesn't exist, at least not in conjunction with having a swimwear body you can be proud of. Every model I have ever met works hard to look great and to keep herself that way. There is no magic, no secret that doctors and nutritionists are hiding from you, despite claims to the contrary. You know the basics—all you need now is a specific plan and a little motivation to make it happen. Part of the motivation comes from KNOWING that you WILL be successful if you follow the program. People don't want to change their diet and avoid the foods they love if, in the end, they're not going to see a noticeable change and hear from their friends that they have changed. So here's my promise to you: Follow our model program for 60 days and you will see a difference…and your friends and family will see it too!

You might think models are immune to such mundane things as cellulite, mommy tummy, and PMS bloat, but that's not true. Models are not some other species of human being with super-powers. They are women just like you, and most of them have to work to maintain their sleek body shape. The battle can seem more challenging as they get older or after they have children. But they do it! Many of our *Venus* models—yes, the ones in the catalogs wearing bikinis—have two or three children, and they come back year after year to model in bikinis again and again! (Physiologically, there is NO reason a woman—including you!—can't stay in great bikini shape well into her 50s or 60s.) In an industry where women over 26 are generally considered "over the hill," most *Venus* models work with us for 10 to 12 years, many into their late 30s. Why? Because *Venus* models value healthy weight loss over starvation…they educate themselves about the foods that can satisfy the body *and* the taste buds…they understand the synergy between diet and exercise…and they start with a healthy base. On those occasions in life when they fall out of shape and have to regain their curves, it is easier—although not a piece of cake, so to speak—because they start with muscle and motivation. Before they begin, they _know_ they will be successful.

> *Model Secret!*
>
> For motivation, I keep a picture on my refrigerator of me when I looked the best I've ever looked in my life. I KNOW I can be that person because that person is me!

We want you to know that you can be successful, too. You just have to think, eat, and act like a *Venus* model. And by the way, our models eat three healthy meals, plus snacks, every day! They never starve themselves, they don't have eating disorders, and they know that being healthy is one of the most important things in the world.

Of course, that doesn't mean that they eat perfectly healthy foods all the time. Everyone—even a supermodel—loosens up on her diet to splurge a little on occasion. The difference is that while many people make eating certain "off-limits" foods a regular thing, models don't sneak treats or indulge in the "bad" foods on a daily (or even weekly) basis. Because models are very aware of their bodies, they tend to have consistently healthy habits. In most cases, they don't give in to momentary whims or cravings. They think long-term. You could say that *they eat with their heads, not their hearts.*

The Venus Summer Shape Up   43

If you follow the principles of healthy eating most of the time, you'll do great. You do not have to forever forego cheeseburgers, but there are guidelines. Let's start with a short (really short!), simple, no-frills lesson in the basics of nutrition. The goal right now is not to make you a food expert, but to give you a general understanding of the terms and concepts that will help you apply the advice given in the rest of this book.

This information is by no means complete—it is bare-bones nutrition so you can get started quickly. You don't have to worry about remembering all of this right now. Later, in section three, we'll tell you exactly which foods to avoid, which to eat, and how much to eat at each sitting. This just gives you some of the reasoning behind our recommendations.

The "Big Three"—Protein, Fat, and Carbohydrates

All food is made up of a combination of three main nutritional components:

1. Protein. The basic building blocks of the muscles, flesh, and other body parts of all animals.

> **Top protein foods:** Animal foods, such as beef, poultry, pork, fish, and seafood. Foods that come from animals, such as milk, cottage cheese, cheese, yogurt, and eggs. Some vegetable foods, such as legumes (black beans, kidney beans, soybeans and tofu, chickpeas), sunflower seeds, nuts, and whole grain breads and cereals.

> **Benefits:** Protein helps keep muscles, bone, hair, and all other body parts strong. It is the most satisfying of the nutrients, helping you feel full more quickly and keeping you from hunger longer.

2. Fats. An important component of cell walls, and a critical ingredient for creating healthy nerve cells and body hormones (and many other things!).

IMPORTANT NOTE: Fats in foods come in different varieties. Eating too many unhealthy fats has been shown to cause heart disease and some cancers. Healthy fats, on the other hand, can help keep your blood vessels clear and are thought to help protect the body from a number of different diseases. The problem is remembering which foods have "good" fats and which have "bad" fats. I'm sure you've heard about saturated, monounsaturated, and polyunsaturated fats. **Saturated fats** are found only in animal foods, and are solid at room temperature. For example, butter and lard are saturated fats. These are generally considered "bad" fats. **Monounsaturated fats** are in liquid form at room temperature, such as olive or canola oil, and are generally considered "good." And **polyunsaturated fats** are a mixed category—some "bad," some "good." There is also a relatively new category called **Trans fats.** These are polyunsaturated fats that have been chemically altered (hydrogenated or partially hydrogenated), and are totally "bad."

> **Best "good" fat foods:** Fish, olive oil, canola oil, avocados, nuts and nut oils, flaxseed and flaxseed oil, sesame seeds and sesame oil.
>
> **WORST "bad" fat foods:** beef (including hamburgers), bacon, butter, stick margarine, whole-fat dairy products (including cheese and ice cream), palm oil, hot dogs, salami, mayonnaise, baked goods with "partially hydrogenated" vegetable oil, crackers, creamy sauces and salad dressings. In addition, bad fats are found in most anything deep-fried, including French fries, funnel cakes (or other fried dough), and fried chicken.
>
> **Benefits:** Cell walls are partially made of fat, so you would completely (and literally) come apart without fats. Fats also help protect and insulate body organs, and store some important vitamins (vitamins A, E, D, and K). Fat is also a good source of long-lasting energy.

3. **Carbohydrates.** Provide quick energy to the body's cells.

IMPORTANT NOTE: As with fats, carbohydrates are not all the same. The more refined the carbohydrate is, the more unhealthy it is. This makes a difference in how you feel physically from minute to minute, hour to hour. It makes a difference in how your body releases and uses insulin, which impacts how quickly and how easily you store fat (or don't). And it makes a difference in how easily you lose weight.

> **Best "good" carbohydrate foods:** Anything made from whole grains, brown rice, quinoa, barley, all fruits (but not fruit juices), legumes, and all vegetables (depending on how they are prepared).

> **WORST "bad" carbohydrate foods:** Sugar, anything made from white flour (including white bread, cakes, cookies, buns, rolls, waffles, pancakes, French toast, bagels, etc).

> **Benefits:** Carbohydrates are a source of quick energy, and some of the good carbs provide important fiber and minerals. The bad carbs, however, are totally unnecessary and serve no healthy purpose whatsoever.

Should You Worry About Vitamins and Minerals?

Worry? No. But it is good to be aware of the nutritional value of what you are eating (and we do recommend that you take a daily multivitamin—more about that later).

Our bodies need vitamins and minerals in order to:

- Make or repair body parts. Example: the mineral calcium, for example, is needed to make bone.

- Help nerves fire correctly so muscles can move. Examples: the minerals calcium and magnesium are used by nerves to help signals reach muscles, and vitamin B6 is important for nerve health.

- Assist body functions; enzymes and hormones couldn't be made without vitamins and minerals, which means that we wouldn't be the people we are without them. Examples: vitamin B12 assists in digestion, vitamin A is important for your eyes, and vitamin C is essential for a good immune system, strong bones and teeth, and healthy skin.

And that's just a portion of everything vitamins and minerals do. Although it would be wonderful if we all ate a perfectly balanced diet, that's not going to happen. Instead, we suggest that you…

1. **Take a multivitamin supplement every day.** This will help make up for any short fall in your diet. (See page 83 for specific recommendations.)

2. **Take calcium supplements daily—500 milligrams, twice a day** (for a total of 1,000 milligrams). It is very difficult to get all the calcium you need from diet alone, so every woman is encouraged to take 1,000 milligrams of calcium each day. Scientists believe the body can absorb no more than about 500 milligrams at a time, so take 500 milligrams in the morning with breakfast, and another 500 milligrams at night with dinner. (See page 83 for specific recommendations.)

3. **Take a cholesterol-free, omega-3 EPA & DHA supplement every day.** These essential fatty acids have been shown to be beneficial for heart health and circulation, allowing optimal levels of oxygen and nutrients to reach your muscles. (See page 83 for specific recommendations.)

4. **Eat a variety of fruits and vegetables.** Each different type of fruit or vegetable contains differing amounts of vitamins, minerals, and a kind of "mini-vitamin" known as phytochemicals. Together, these elements keep you healthy, help prevent diseases (including cancer!), make you strong, improve your mood, and help your body use the energy it gets

from food. Phytochemicals are a relatively new discovery. There are thousands of them, and more are being discovered every day. Obviously, you won't be able to keep track of them, so the trick is to eat many different kinds of fruits and vegetables so you take in all the nutrition you can. For example, although broccoli is good for you, if you eat it every day, you'll miss out on the phytochemicals it doesn't have. That's why you should try to mix it up a bit. Broccoli today, spinach tomorrow, squash on Friday—you get the picture.

If you do just those four things, you'll be better off nutritionally than probably 90 percent of the population.

CALORIES!!!

The diet industry goes through its own fashion transitions—"low-fat" turns into "no-carb," which gives way to "high-protein," which swings into "fasting and cleansing." While each has merits, most are really just the fad *du jour*.

The fashion industry thrives on finding the latest colors, textures, and styles. Fashion is part art, part architecture, and part whimsy. Nutrition is NONE of those things. The human body does not change quite so dramatically, although our understanding of how it works seems to change almost hourly.

Weight loss fads come from frustration. A lot of women ask themselves, "Why didn't that last diet work for me?" Of course, the next logical thought is that maybe, just maybe, the next one will work better, so they grab on to the latest big diet kick (or worse, the latest "miracle pill") like it is the last remaining life-vest in a sinking boat. Here's the interesting thing, proved by medical researchers: All diets lead to weight loss, and the amount of loss from diet to diet does not vary widely, but recent studies have shown that eating proteins and avoiding carbs is the best way to shed fat. Without carbs available as fuel, the body is forced to burn fat stores. Bodybuilders have to shed almost all fat—they get down to 3% to 5% body fat at competition time—and they do that by avoiding carbs. We provide a very low-carb diet because it's not just less weight we want—it's that we want MORE muscle and LESS fat as well. Building muscle is just as essential as losing fat. (We'll talk more about why this is essential later.) To build that muscle, we need lots of protein, and we need to limit the carbs we take in so we can force the body to burn fat—the excess fat you are carrying—for its fuel.

But before we get to the specifics of the diet let's discuss some basics:

What is a calorie?

A calorie is simply a way to measure the energy we get from food. Some foods give us more energy than others, and these are said to have more "calories." It's important to say here that we're not talking about "energy" in the everyday sense of the word, where you might say, "I had more energy than I thought, so I walked an extra mile." Energy from calories is more like fuel.

But calories are not all alike.

The idea of "calorie" as a standard unit of energy was created by scientists, and the number of calories you read on a label for a given food were determined in a laboratory. But weight control is not just about calories that you eat; how your body processes the different types of food is important too. Your body is not a laboratory furnace! Different kinds of calories can prompt your body to do different things. With each mouthful of food you eat, your body has to mobilize a complex system to digest, absorb, and use each of the nutrients…and the reaction your body has to the types of food you eat causes different physiological reactions. That's why a calorie isn't always a calorie!

Carbohydrate energy burns the fastest. It provides immediate fuel for the body. If your body has carbs to burn, it will burn them BEFORE it starts to use your fat stores as energy. I met an aerobic instructor who taught 3 classes a day, 6 days a week and she was still 30 pounds overweight. She didn't understand why she couldn't lose weight when she was literally spending 3 hours per day doing aerobics –that's a lot of exercise! The answer was really quite simple. To teach her class, she felt she needed immediate energy and so, prior to **each** class, she would eat a high carb meal or snack. Her favorite was a bowl of Raisin Bran (almost all carbs) with 2% milk. Well, one bowl of her "energy food" contains 300 calories—and in an hour of aerobics, you burn about 300 calories. So in 5 minutes she could easily consume as many calories as she would burn off in a full hour of aerobics! Sure, she had plenty of energy, but there was NO net loss. Her body was burning the Raisin Bran for her fuel source instead of burning the excess fat she really wanted to get rid of. Had she done the aerobics without all those carbs in her system, she would have forced her body to turn to the next available energy source (fat) as fuel for her classes, and she would have lost weight.

There is an important point here: You cannot exercise your way out of a bad diet! Burning calories through exercise takes a LOT longer than it takes to consume those same calories. One wrong meal might give you 10 minutes of pleasure, but to get rid of that meal you will likely have to spend 1 or 2 hours in the gym. It's a tough equation, but it's true. Exercise is HUGELY important, but, for maximum results, you must combine that with a careful diet.

Have you ever seen little kids wired on sugar? They run, flail, jump, yell, turn circles, and generally act goofy until the sugar "wears off," and then they crash. That's sort of how your body reacts to carbs—it feels the energy rush, your blood sugar spikes, and your body revs up and prepares to process the energy. This process involves releasing lots of insulin, and insulin is the "storage hormone." Insulin takes any excess carbs you don't burn up right away and turns them into body fat. You'll find those carbs later in the mirror! Just as quickly your blood sugar falls and you are left feeling sluggish and exhausted. Carbohydrates from whole grains cause a less dramatic sugar spike because the fiber in those "good" carbs slows the release of insulin, evening out the highs and lows and making it less likely your body will store them as fat. Complex carbs cause an insulin release too; it's just not as rapid or extreme.

Calorie energy from fat burns much more slowly than calorie energy from carbs. Of the three major nutrients, protein is the most diet-friendly. It is difficult to process, which means that your body actually uses more energy processing protein than it does processing carbs or fats. So eating 100 calories worth of protein REALLY gives your body fewer net calories (due to the energy cost of digesting proteins) than does eating 100 calories worth of carbs which takes almost no energy to process. To summarize bluntly: *Carbs set your body up to store fat,* so they need to be chosen carefully and eaten in limited quantities; proteins *set your body up to lose fat* because they burn more calories, help you build muscle (in conjunction with training), and raise metabolism. Fats go along for the ride.

Model Secret!

Keep a log! Few people realize how much they really eat. For just one week, carry a little spiral notebook with you and write down EVERY-THING you put into your mouth. Get a calorie book from any book store and add it up. You will likely find that you are consuming far more calories than you think you are. And really seeing and understanding what you are eating—seeing it before you in black and white—can provide motivation to change.

The *Venus Summer Shape Up* gives you the right combination of carbohydrates, fats, and proteins to ensure a good energy balance and the nutrition you need to stay healthy and strong. We use an actual equation to calculate which foods you should eat at each meal based on the percentage of calories from each of the different food components we want you to consume. We did it so you don't have to. The diet that begins on page 79 takes all these factors into account and tells you exactly what to eat and when to eat it. We also tell you how much to eat! So while you can count calories if you wish, it isn't necessary on our program. Our diet (with portion sizes) will help control your total calorie intake, and our bias toward proteins will ensure that the calories you do eat actually help you to build muscle and lose fat. This is important because, although calories are not all equal, you simply cannot eat all you want. The amount of food you eat (as well as the type of food) minus what you burn each day determines whether you gain or lose weight.

The Truth about Weight Loss

Remember the episode of *I Love Lucy* where Lucy and Ethel get jobs packaging chocolates at a candy factory? At first, the candies come rolling down the conveyor belt at a nice, slow pace, and the women have no trouble placing each chocolate neatly in a box. Soon, the belt speeds up, and more and more chocolates need boxing, but the women can't keep up. They collect chocolates in their aprons, stuff them down their blouses, and stuff their mouths full, all in a futile attempt to get rid of the excess candy that just keeps coming down the belt.

That's a great image for what happens with calories and weight gain. Imagine that the chocolates represent calories. The basic fact is this:

If you can't "get rid" of calories fast enough, they start to accumulate. And as calories accumulate, you gain weight.

If you have gained weight in the past year or the past 5 years, you have simply consumed more calories than you have used. It really is just that simple.

When calories accumulate, your body stores them as fat—the kind that settles around your waist, hips, or thighs. If you collect 3,500 extra calories, you put on a pound of body weight. Those "extra" calories represent the chocolates that came down the conveyor belt that Lucy couldn't get rid of. Every day, your body gets rid of calories with every little thing that requires energy, from mindless activities like breathing and growing your fingernails, to conscious movement, such as walking up the stairs, driving, playing tennis, or any other activity. That's what people mean when they talk about "burning" calories. The more you do, the more calories you burn.

In a perfect world, the number of calories you eat every day would exactly match the number of calories you burn. Eat a cookie, burn a cookie's worth of energy, and everything would stay the same—no weight gained, no weight lost. What usually happens, however, is that you burn a cookie's worth of energy, but eat three cookies—or more. All those extra calories accumulate and get turned into body weight, and sadly, that weight is usually fat.

Model Secret!

Alcohol contains a lot of calories that many people don't count. Did you know that, ounce-for-ounce, wine contains three times as many calories as a light beer? A 12-ounce light beer contains about 90 calories, and a 4-ounce glass of wine also contains 90 calories. (Of course, most servings of wine are far more than 4 ounces. According to one study, a typical serving is closer to 120 calories.) A standard martini with an olive contains about 180 calories, and a Cosmopolitan contains 151 calories. Oh, and by the way, a slice of cheese pizza contains about 180 calories. So every time you have an 8-ounce glass of wine or a mixed drink, you might as well be eating a slice of pizza! If you drink just ONE mixed drink, or two light beers, or two 4-ounce glasses of wine per day (one standard 8-ounce glass), in one year you will have consumed 65,700 calories! That's enough extra calories to add up to a weight gain of 18 pounds PER YEAR that would not be there if you did NOTHING other than eliminate the beer or the alcohol!

BUT...the reverse also happens. If you eat fewer calories than you burn, you lose weight! Your body takes calories out of storage by breaking down body fat (or muscle) and turning it back into energy to provide fuel for your activities. Because we want to lose the fat, not the muscle, workouts (which preserve muscle) are extremely important. So, if you want to lose weight, you can, of course, eat less. This would be like having fewer chocolates come down the conveyor belt so Lucy can handle them easily. You can also lose weight by burning more calories, which you can do by becoming more active with exercise. This would be like having Lucy move faster so none of the chocolates got by her. You also have a third option—you can turn up your personal heat, also known as your basal metabolism, so you can burn more calories in the same amount of time. In our Lucy example, this would be as if Lucy had suddenly cloned herself so she didn't have to work as hard and could still stay on top of the chocolate situation. (Okay, that's enough talk about chocolates!)

Mastering Metabolism

You know how some women seem to be able to eat anything and not gain an ounce? Do they have something you don't? Well...yeah. (Sorry.) Everyone is born with a certain inborn, genetic metabolism, the rate at which she is able to use calories. Some people just burn a little "hotter" on the inside. They are energy inefficient, like a human version of the gas-guzzling Hummer—they need a lot more fuel to go a mile than other cars need. Low-metabolism people, on the other hand, conserve fuel like a Prius hybrid. The problem is that what's good for cars is a real problem for people. In people, conserving energy means it is easier to accumulate calories and put on body fat.

If only there were a way to raise your metabolism.... But wait! There is! In fact, there are two ways: 1) the food burn, and 2) the muscle burn.

The basic physiology of the human body hasn't changed since the days of the cavemen (and cavewomen!). Back then, they didn't have traditional, sit-down, three-times-per-day meals. They were hunters and gatherers. In times when they had a lot of food, they ate throughout the day, grazing on small meals. They ate often and maintained a feeling of being satisfied—not stuffed, not starved, but just right. In this state of having enough food, the body sent hormone signals that said, in effect, "I'm being fed frequently, so

I don't need to be storing fat; there's always more food coming." In the winters when food was scarce, our ancestors ate once a day (if they were lucky). The body's reaction was to automatically go into starvation mode by ratcheting down metabolism so that it could store whatever was being consumed. This was a good thing back then, and people who were fortunate enough to have a slow metabolism (and therefore packed on fat more easily) were able to survive when their faster-burning friends starved to death.

Unfortunately, our bodies still do that! If you eat one meal a day—and it doesn't matter if that meal is huge—all the body knows is that it is being fed only once a day, and it does the same thing it did in caveman days: it ratchets down your metabolism, prepares for starvation, and starts storing fat. Your body doesn't know when the next meal is coming, so it reacts accordingly. Doctors see patients all the time who come in and say, "I don't understand how I can be gaining weight (or not losing weight)—I eat only once a day!" Well, it's all about metabolism. Our bodies still respond in those pre-programmed ways, and they don't know or care that you can make a single phone call and have pizza delivered to your door virtually any time of the day. When our bodies sense an impending famine because they are not fed regularly, our metabolism slows to conserve fuel just as it did in prehistoric times. To our bodies, "famine" can mean anything from missing breakfast to going too long between meals, to going on a starvation diet.

While this may seem counterintuitive, you have to keep the "food burn" going strong by convincing your body that there's plenty of food coming and there is no need for it to slow down your metabolism and start storing fat. To do this, it is important to:

- **Always eat breakfast.** Breakfast gives your body the energy it needs to function well during the day, and it warms up a metabolism that has been on a slow idle all night while you were sleeping. People who eat breakfast keep their metabolism running higher and hotter than it would if they skipped that meal.

- **Eat three meals a day, AND eat two snacks daily.** Just as breakfast warms up your daily metabolism, eating regularly—about every two to three hours—keeps your metabolism fires stoked. Later, in chapter 8, we'll tell you exactly what and how much to eat at each meal and snack. Although you want to eat frequently, you don't want to eat too much.

- **Don't starve.** A lot of women believe that the longer they can hold off until eating, the less they will eat all day, and therefore they will lose weight faster. That has two major flaws—they are actually more likely to lose weight if they eat breakfast (and spark their metabolism), and starving just lowers the metabolism, making it even harder to lose weight. Long-term dieters eventually find that they have to eat less and less food to maintain their weight, which means they starve more, lowering their metabolism further still, and getting progressively more miserable as they try to eat less and less, fighting their bodies each step of the way. That's a diet doomed to failure.

> *Model Secret!*
>
> Models typically "graze" throughout the day instead of stuffing themselves at one major meal per day. Eating frequent small meals is one of the major keys to success.

The overall metabolism message is that food is good for you! The right foods are nutritious, they give you energy, and they help your metabolism kick in and burn hotter and longer. That's why it is important not to skip any of the meals or snacks we list in the meal plans. And it is also why we can assure you that, on The *Venus Summer Shape Up Program,* **you will not starve!** On this program, eating—and eating *well*—is a top priority.

Your next priority is to master the second method of raising your metabolism for faster weight loss: the "muscle burn." It is so important that we devote the entire next chapter to it.

Chapter 5:
Movement 101

For many people, exercise feels like punishment, something unpleasant to be avoided whenever possible. If that sounds like you, we're going to spend this chapter helping you to "reframe" the way you think about activity, movement, and work-outs.

"Reframing" is a psychological technique that helps people feel better about a situation simply by changing how they think about it. For example, women who have a hard time getting over a bad break-up might be encouraged to reframe the experience. Instead of getting stuck on the break-up feelings of sadness and rejection, they could change their focus to one of appreciation for all the extra time they have to spend with other friends. This change of attitude doesn't happen in a flash—it takes time and practice. But just as walking the same route through a forest will eventually wear a clear pathway, thinking the same thoughts—even if you don't necessarily believe them right away—will eventually cause your mind to take that familiar path in the future. In other words, if you think enough positive thoughts about exercise, you might eventually have positive feelings about exercise! You just have to get over the negativity hurdle.

Feeling good about exercise is important because there is really no way around it. No pill you can take will give you lasting weight loss, and diet alone will seldom lead to long-term weight loss or the results you want. Exercise in addition to diet really is the only "quick fix" there is. Here are some of the benefits you can keep in mind as you reframe your feelings about working out:

- Exercise generates energy.

- Exercise turns your body into a fat-burning machine.

- Exercise makes you feel good, both physically and mentally.

- Exercise makes you physically and mentally strong.

- Exercise helps all your body parts function better, so you reduce your risk of long-term diseases, especially heart disease—the biggest killer of women overall. In addition, exercise can help you manage or reduce symptoms of most other chronic diseases, including autoimmune disorders, diabetes, irritable bowel syndrome (IBS), insomnia, and tension headaches.

- Exercise improves mood and reduces anxiety.

- Exercise improves your ability to handle stress and reduces physical stress reactions.

- Exercise can improve or eliminate symptoms of premenstrual syndrome (PMS).

- Exercise seems to increase the body's levels of natural "feel-good" chemicals, including endorphins and phenylethylamine. Endorphins are the body's version of morphine; they can reduce pain and cause a sense of euphoria. Endorphins are considered to be a major cause of the well-known "runner's high." Phenylethylamine is another chemical compound that helps make us feel happy. How happy? Phenylethylamine is also found in chocolate and is thought to be the reason so many women are drawn to chocolate when they feel that they need a pick-me-up. So exercise is better than chocolate—all the joy, none of the weight gain.

Two Kinds of Fun...

Exercise has two main purposes: 1) burning calories *right now* (as you exercise) so you get rid of some of your body fat, and 2) raising your basal metabolism so you burn more calories overall – even when you're resting! When you have a higher metabolic rate, you become one of those women who look like they never have to worry about their weight—you can eat more and still lose weight.

Your metabolism is determined by structures in your cells called mitochondria. These are the power-packs of the body, capable of turning calories and oxygen into energy. To raise your metabolism, you need to either increase the number of mitochondria you have or improve the mitochondria's oxygen—calorie burn rate. Or both! The only way to accomplish all this calorie-burning, metabolism-raising, weight-loss perfection is to make a habit of two different kinds of exercise—aerobic movement and strength training.

Model Secret!

It is impossible to spot-reduce. Your body decides where to store fat. Some people store it around their waists; others store it around their hips and thighs. When your body burns fat, it burns it first from the LAST place you stored it. If you tend to store fat in your thighs first and your stomach second, you can do leg lifts all day long, but you won't lose thigh fat until the stomach fat is gone! If you focus on losing weight IN GENERAL, it will all come off eventually.

Aerobic movement

Aerobic exercise is any type of movement that increases your need for oxygen because you continue a moderate effort over a relatively long period of time. Examples include walking, running, swimming and cycling.

You know yourself, from the amount of huffing and puffing you experience while performing these types of exercises, that aerobic movement requires oxygen. This means that aerobic exercise works to raise metabolism by increasing your cell's oxygen—calorie burn rate. But that's only half the story. Muscles that work hard have more mitochondria. For example, cells in the heart are packed with mitochondria. When you work your body's muscles, you can increase the mitochondria in those cells. That's an automatic boost in fat-burning ability.

That's why half your exercise routine involves aerobic movement and half involves strength training. We'll tell you exactly what exercise to do, when to do it, and for how long.

Model Secret!

If you don't feel great—physically or emotionally—don't cancel your workout! Going through the motions and doing something (anything) on those "down" days is better than doing nothing at all. Maintain the habit!

Strength training

Strength training is anaerobic, which means that it doesn't require as much oxygen. Anaerobic exercises—such as doing push-ups, lifting a dumbbell, or pulling on a resistance band--involve short bursts of energy and exertion. Strength training raises your metabolism by increasing your muscle mass, and the more muscle you have, the more mitochondria you have, and the more calories you burn all day long. In The *Venus Summer Shape Up,* half your exercise time will be devoted to building muscles with strength training.

I know some of you are thinking: "Muscles?!? Who wants muscles?" Many women are worried about building too much muscle because they are afraid they will look less feminine, or they will somehow burst out of their clothes like the Incredible Hulk. Actually, you have a better chance of bursting out of your clothes if you **don't** exercise! The only way a woman can put on the kind of muscle that begins to look masculine is if she injects herself with testosterone, the natural male hormone (or other illegal anabolic steroids). The average woman cannot possibly put on unattractive amounts of muscle. Let's make that perfectly clear:

Working out with weights will not make you look like a professional wrestler!

It just cannot happen. What building muscle does (aside from raising your metabolism) is help make your body more compact and defined. Fat is lost. Muscles tighten. You'll fit into that bikini you've been dying to wear, and you'll probably need to buy a whole new wardrobe of smaller clothes.

Muscles also help to reduce the signs of aging: You'll get older, but you'll look better at every age. People talk about their metabolism slowing as they get older, but most of it is totally controllable. About 95 percent of the apparent "slowing" of metabolism that so many people use as the excuse for gaining weight as they age IS NOT because of the endless parade of birthdays, but because we have less muscle than we had when we were younger. And why is that? Well, most of us are less active than we were when we were in our teens or 20s—much less active. Less activity means less muscle, which means a slower metabolism. When you do strength training, you can offset most of that muscle loss and keep your metabolism at its highest level. You can look spectacular today, next year, and when you are 75! Keeping your muscle mass is the key, and strength training is the ONLY way to accomplish that.

Model Secret!

Ninety percent of our *Venus* models do some sort of strength training or weight lifting <u>in</u> addition to their aerobic workouts. NINETY PERCENT!

Muscle Burn

In order to improve your "muscle burn" and keep it (and you) hot, you need to:

- **Follow the program.** In your enthusiasm, you may be tempted to do more than the recommended amount of exercise. Don't. It's easy to over-do it and burn out if you try to do it all at once. The program moves you up the Phase levels slowly so you ease into a good exercise routine.

- **Be aware of the good "sore" from a good workout vs "hurt".** When you exercise muscles you haven't used much (at least not lately), the usual result is some soreness—a kind of deep, mild ache in the muscles. This is normal and natural and a good thing. It's a sign that you're doing good work. In a couple of days, the soreness goes away. (You can always take an over-the-counter pain reliever if you normally do so for headaches and such.) The pain of an injury is very different. If you feel sharp pain, pain in a joint, or pain that feels unbearable, stop what you're doing! If the pain continues, see a doctor. Be wise about the signals your body is giving you.

- **Find your groove.** Are you a morning person or a night owl? Do you have trouble sleeping, or do you need help waking up? We all have different times to work out that are optimal for us. Some people like to exercise first thing in the morning to make sure it gets done no matter what else happens during the day. Others prefer to exercise after work as a way to unwind after a long day. Or maybe you can take an extra half hour to exercise before lunch. Find the time that works best for you—but definitely find the time.

Model Secret!

If you can afford it, hire a personal trainer for a couple of months to help you get started and to keep you motivated. If you can't afford or can't find a personal trainer, recruit a friend to join you on your quest for a better body! If you know someone is going to meet you for a workout at a specified time, you are less likely to skip the workout. Find an accountability partner!

The exercises outlined in the Program are necessary to help raise your metabolism and lose weight. But we encourage you to stay as active as possible beyond the guidelines of the Program. Go dancing…learn to surf…hike in the mountains…try kayaking…take a yoga class…bike with your kids. Anything fun that gets your body moving will enhance your experience with the Program. This could be the start of a whole new life.

Chapter 6:

A Model Story—Rachel

Rachel is sweet, smart, and quietly poetic. Although she has been modeling for only five years, she is already a national sensation because of her work as a model on *The Price is Right.*

I wish I could just roll out of bed and look fabulous. I always have to "worry" about my body. I try to eat healthy, but I'm not always the healthiest eater. My close friends know I don't follow an ideal diet all the time. For me, it is easier to manage my shape with exercise than with food. If I have a photo shoot coming up, I'll get very strict prior to the shoot—no sweet stuff. But if I don't have to get into a bikini anytime soon, I'll eat things that I KNOW are bad for me. I'm not too careful, but I never let my eating get me too far out of shape—I can never tell when the phone will ring and I have to be ready to shoot on very short notice.

I don't believe in starving myself to lose weight—it's not fun, and it's not healthy. I have to eat breakfast within 15 minutes of waking up. I've gotten sick from not eating breakfast. Other than that, I don't really do anything special with my diet, but I don't eat large volumes of food. Exercise is a different story. I love to work out. The reason I don't have to worry about my diet so much is because I maintain my fitness.

I work out at least 5 days per week, sometimes more. I do 50 minutes of cardio…then 20 minutes of crunches, push-ups, and some free weights…and I end with about 30 minutes of stretching. I take my time—I don't rush through my workout. It may not sound like much time, but I work out really hard. When I'm done with my 50 minutes of cardio, I'm sweating so much I look like I just showered with my clothes on. I love to work on my stomach with crunches and this exercise where I hang from a bar and do leg lifts (I love that one). I also do a lot of lunges while holding free weights. I like to use weight machines to do leg extensions and leg curls. By the way, when I use machines, I do one leg at a time. I find that if I use both legs simultaneously, the results can be uneven if one leg compensates for weakness in the other. Of course, I go in spurts with what I do on any given day. Lately, push-ups are my thing.

I also enjoy running. I ran track through high school and for Louisiana State University. I'll run on a treadmill if I have to, but I prefer running outside on a track. Some people find it boring, but I like it. I've been running on a track since I was 13 years old. You know how a soccer player might enjoy the smell of a fresh-mowed lawn? I like the smell of a track! I'm comfortable there. When I run on a track, I don't have to think about getting hit by a car. I can let my mind go; not think about it. Plus, a track often has the rubber surface which cushions your joints and ankles.

My "tricks"

The most important thing to remember is that when you start on a new fitness program, your muscles are going to be sore in the beginning. A lot of people are surprised when that happens and get discouraged, but it is perfectly normal, and it's a good thing. It tells you that what you are doing is working! That soreness is your muscles' response to the exercise. It's breaking down and building more muscle, and that's just what you want. Just remember that your first goal is just to get through that first month. After that, working out feels good, and it starts to turn into a habit (a good habit!) and you don't ever get as sore as when you first started. It really does get easier. I was fortunate to have fitness in my life from the time I was very young. Now, when I feel that little muscle ache, I know it means I've done something good for my body. It's a sign of getting stronger. The hurt and ache you get a day or two after a workout is very different from the sharp pain of a muscle pull or ligament tear. If you have sharp pain, see a doctor!

I realize that sometimes it's hard for women to exercise on a regular basis. People tend to get bored doing the same thing everyday. Well, my advice is that you don't have to stick to the same regimen day in and day out. Have fun with your workout! Change it up. If you are a good swimmer, then swim in a pool for your workout. If you like the outdoors, go out for a run or a hike. If you prefer air conditioning, run on a treadmill or work out on an elliptical machine at the gym. And I haven't even mentioned bike riding, rowing, yoga, tennis—there are so many different ways to stay fit. Do what you like; what feels best for your body, but do something! Everyone is different. Plus, when you change your routine, you use different muscle groups each time.

Now, let's say you do suffer a minor injury--you tweak a knee, pull a calf muscle, or twist an ankle. The most important thing is to NOT completely stop working out when you have an injury. If you stop, you risk getting out of the groove of working out. My advice? Just don't work that particular injured area. Stay active—there is always something else you can do that won't bother your injury. For example, just a few months ago I pulled my left calf muscle, so instead of running (which I most enjoy), I rode a stationary bike. And I even changed that up with a few workouts on the elliptical every other day. Another important thing you can do for yourself during an injury is to slowly stretch the injured area daily. Stretching can help the injured area heal faster. These should be long, slow, easy stretches—NOT the bouncy,

Model Secret!

I keep a stack of catalogs and magazines at hand that I look through periodically. When I see the other models' bodies, it motivates me to stay in shape.

jerky stretches some people tend to do. If you don't stretch while healing there is a greater possibility that the area could get re-injured. Now, I'm no doctor, but I've learned these simple solutions thanks to my trainers when I used to run track at Louisiana State University.

My final "trick" is really simple: DRINK WATER! In the past year, I've had only about one soft drink—and I used to drink them every single day. It was a hard habit to break, but I did it! I started drinking water instead, and I've noticed a big difference. Water makes me feel "moisturized" inside and out. Water feeds your muscles, so workouts are easier, and you'll be less likely to cramp up. My skin looks better, too. Plus, soft drinks have a lot of calories. By substituting water for soda, I'm not gaining weight from the extra calories. I'm a water believer.

Living this kind of active lifestyle is not only good for you as an individual, but it is good for your family, too. Fitness is catching. If you do it, your children will look at you as a role model, as I did my parents. They will grow up healthy and strong, and fitness will be a regular part of their lives. With fitness in your life, it can be a long, happy, healthy life in which you always look fabulous!

Rachel's model secrets…

- Doesn't believe in starving herself.

- Eats breakfast within 15 minutes of waking up.

- Looks at pictures of other models in magazines for inspiration.

- Water is an important part of her health regimen.

- Loves working out.

- Works out 5 days per week. Does 50 minutes of cardio, 20 minutes of strength training, and 30 minutes of stretching. Loves running, especially on a track.

- Understands that good health is a habit, and that exercise needs to be fun.

Section Three

The Venus Summer
Shape Up

Chapter 7:
GETTING STARTED!

The *Venus Summer Shape Up* has three phases:

Phase 1—Wake-Up Call

Phase 2—Transformation

Phase 3—Energizing

Each phase lasts 20 days, and each has a **Food Plan** and an **Exercise Program.**

FOOD PLAN

The Food Plan is toughest in Phase 1, but it gets more lenient as you proceed to Phase 2 and Phase 3. We do this to get your body into fat-burning mode as quickly as possible.

It takes about 2 to 4 weeks for the body to get into a fat-burning mode. Think of it like trying to start a car that has been sitting in the driveway for a month—it may take a little while for the engine to turn over...the battery might have died...and there's a warm-up period before the car is ready to roar down the street. Your body has been idle, and you need to jump your battery and crank your starter (so to speak). After 2 to 4 weeks, your body will have "learned" that it isn't facing starvation so it is okay to start burning calories, and your muscles will have developed to a point where your natural metabolism will be higher than before you started.

During those 2 to 4 weeks, your body will resist change as it tries to figure out what's going on. During that time, you won't see any dramatic early weight loss. Once your body is a fat-burning machine, the weight will start to fall off. We recommend that, after your initial weigh-in, you don't get back on a scale until after 30 days have passed—when you are in the middle of Phase 2. Instead of relying on the scale to validate your efforts, trust that it is working. Notice that your jeans might be looser, and enjoy the extra energy you'll have from eating well and working out.

To give you a little extra motivation, we've built a *Free Day* into the program. Here's how it works: If you follow the program for six days **with no cheats on food or exercise**, then the seventh day is your *Free Day*, during which you can eat whatever foods you like during that day's meals. (NOTE: This is not an excuse to pig out! This freedom means you can eat regular meal-sized portions of your choice of foods. Also, there are foods you should not <u>ever</u> have because they are not merely unhealthy, they are toxic to your body. You'll find a list of these foods in chapter 8.) You will probably find that the foods you used to love become less appealing over time, and your desire for them will fade. Soon, the *Free Day* won't feel like a big deal because the foods on the diet will have become the foods you love.

Food Plan Tips

1. *Learn to read food labels.* If you are going to eat healthy, you have to know what ingredients are in the packaged foods you buy.

2. *ELIMINATE any food that contains high fructose corn syrup.* Researchers are discovering that many of our weight problems can be traced to high quantities of a sweetener called high fructose corn syrup (let's call it HFCS for short). It's in a lot of foods you probably have on your shelf, including some packaged baked goods, soups, sauces, cereals, and on and on. Read the labels of anything you buy, and do not buy anything with HFCS. Think of it as a toxin to your body—one that causes extra body fat—and avoid it as if it were rat poison.

3. *Always eat breakfast.* It really is the most important meal of the day because it provides energy and sparks metabolism.

4. *Don't skip meals.* We want to keep your metabolism going by letting your body know that there is a steady supply of good food coming. So don't skip the planned meals or snacks.

5. *Drink water.* You should drink a glass of water 15 minutes prior to every meal. This will help ensure you are getting the water you need and will help you to feel full faster when you do eat. We also recommend that you drink water as your beverage with your meal.

6. *Eat dinner early.* We recommend eating dinner no later than 7:00 pm. The stomach takes 2 to 3 hours to empty, and you shouldn't go to bed with food in your stomach. If you must eat later because of your work schedule, eat a smaller portion.

7. *Don't eat extra when you feel stressed.* Comfort foods are weight-gain foods. If you need to vent stress, exercise instead.

8. *Hide the big plates and bowls.* Most people eat with their eyes as much as with their stomachs. They fill their plates and eat until every morsel is gone. You know that you shouldn't clean your plate, but it is difficult not to. That's why we recommend using smaller plates and bowls for your food. Instead of the dinner plate, use the smaller size—the salad or luncheon plate. Your eyes will see a full plate, your stomach won't get stuffed, you'll maintain control over food portions, but you'll still feel satisfied!

9. *Leave the room during food commercials.* Watching too much TV is a risk factor for weight gain, so we recommend that you cut back on the amount of time you spend sitting and watching. (Of course, if you have the TV on while you're on the treadmill, that's a positive

use of the technology!) But what's worse is that the food commercials are so pervasive and destructive. If it is advertised, chances are it is full of bad fats, cheese, and sugar. They are in our faces all day long, and some people are very susceptible to the messages. Don't give them a chance to sabotage your diet—close your eyes, mute the sound, leave the room.

EXERCISE PROGRAM

The Exercise Program starts out easy in Phase 1 and becomes progressively more difficult in Phase 2 and Phase 3. We know it is difficult to start a new exercise program if you've been inactive for awhile. That's why we start out easy. (Well, not too easy. We're still going to make you sweat.) The Phase 1 Wake-Up Call exercise program is designed for BEGINNERS. Phase 2 is INTERMEDIATE, and Phase 3 is for ADVANCED exercisers only.

If you are already active, feel free to move up to Phase 2. If that's too easy, try the Phase 3 exercise program. (If you skip exercise levels, do not skip the food levels!)

Our exercise program has two different tracks—one for people who have access to a gym, and one for people who don't. For each weight training exercise, you'll find instructional photographs of one of our *Venus* models performing the steps, as well as a full description of the proper form.

Exercise Program Tips

1. *If possible, find a partner.* A partner can help motivate you, encourage you, and get you moving on days when you don't feel like exercising. A partner can also watch to make sure you are doing the exercises with proper form, without straining or otherwise risking injury.

74   The Venus Summer Shape Up

2. ***Remember, we're talking about half an hour.*** Our exercise program is condensed—starting with just 30 minutes once or twice a day. When you think you don't have time to work-out, remember that we're talking about half the time it takes to watch an episode of *Grey's Anatomy*! You **must** have 30 minutes you can devote to pampering yourself with the promise of a better body.

3. ***Work out for AT LEAST one minute.*** We all have days when we don't feel like working out. Don't just plop on the couch. Instead, get dressed in your work-out clothes and do the day's routine for at least one minute. Trainers know that it is often the first minute that's difficult— the next 29 minutes are easy. Exercise generates energy, immediately and long-term. Most people who begin an exercise session end up finishing their routine…the trick is taking that first step.

START HERE...

- **Ask a friend to help you take "before" pictures of yourself.** Wear a swimsuit and get four good shots: one from the front, one from behind, and one from each side.

- **Weigh yourself.** Write your weight on the Progress Chart located on page 78 next to *Starting Weight*.

- **Take your physical measurements.** Using a flexible tape measure, measure your waist, hips, and thighs. (The hip measurement should be taken at the widest part of your lower body. The thigh measurement should be taken halfway between your knee and your crotch. The waist measurement should be taken at the smallest part of your middle, or about an inch above your bellybutton.) Record these numbers on the Progress Chart on page 78.

- **Make a promise...**NOT to weigh or measure yourself, OR look at the Progress Chart again until after you have completed 30 days of the program.

- **Post your inspiration.** In chapter 2, you defined your personal weight loss goal—your "Beach." Using whatever sources you want, find or create a representation of your goal. You can cut a picture out of a magazine, find an old photograph, write words on a piece of paper in bold marker, use a souvenir from a meaningful place, or anything else that will scream at you when you look at it. Post it someplace where you are likely to see it often—the bathroom mirror, the front door, next to the treadmill, above the TV. By posting your goal, you are giving yourself a visual reminder of why you have begun this adventure in healthy living.

- **Get rid of temptation.** You know which foods are your favorite cravings or binge foods. Dump them! Go through the kitchen and make sure it is a junk-free zone…and keep it that way! If you buy your favorite food to eat on your *"Free Day,"* chuck whatever is left over into the garbage before the next diet day begins. And it's not going to hurt the rest of your family to eat healthfully either!

- **Remember that The *Venus Summer Shape Up* is primarily about creating a healthy lifestyle.** Although we are using the word "diet," that word implies that you simply stop after you reach your goal. That's how yo-yo weight gain and loss happen. The goal is to lose the weight, reach your Beach, and then stay there by continuing the program. Our models don't stop thinking about their diet and health once the cameras stop shooting—they know that life goes on even after the photographer goes home. We hope you make this program a permanent part of your life.

TO THE BEACH!

Starting Date: _8/20/2012_

    Switch to Phase 2: _____

    Switch to Phase 3: _____

End Date: _____

Starting Weight: _128_

Starting Measurements:

    Waist: _30_

    Hips: _36_

    Thigh: _31.5_

End Weight: _____

End Measurements:

    Waist: _____

    Hips: _____

    Thigh: _____

Subtract end weight from starting weight to get total pounds lost. _____

Subtract end measurements from starting measurements to get _____
the number of inches lost.

Chapter 8:
Eat Like a Model—
3 Phases of Food

When most people think about going on a "diet," they think only about eating less. Instead of two Big Macs, they eat just one, or instead of a big plate of spaghetti and meatballs, they have just the spaghetti. That's half of a good idea. With The *Venus Summer Shape Up*, we ask you to eat *normal portion sizes,* which may be less—or, in some cases more—than what you are eating now, AND to focus on *foods that promote fat loss,* as opposed to foods that encourage fat storage.

Real weight loss occurs only by eating the right foods in the right portions, and combining that with appropriate exercise.

Eating like a model is probably going to seem quite foreign to you. It is a different way of thinking about food. Like athletes and other professionals whose bodies are centrally important to their lives, models know that food is NOT a treat, or an indulgence, or a safety blanket, or a form of entertainment. Food is fuel. Food is energy, vitamins, minerals, and other nutrients. Food is NOT your enemy; it is the most powerful ally you have in getting healthy in the body you want.

The trick is knowing which foods to eat, which ones to avoid, and how and when to eat the foods that will help you achieve your goals. Keeping your goal in mind is key. You must truly believe that success is possible and that the program WILL work. Always keep your goal in mind and understand that this is THE path that will lead you to your goal.

The *Venus Summer Shape Up* Food Plan

Each phase of The *Venus Summer Shape Up* program lasts 20 days. We recommend that everyone start with Phase One.

The food plan itself is simple. We give you a list of approved foods, clustered into broad nutrient categories: Proteins, Complex Carbohydrates, Fruits and Vegetables, Beverages, Snacks, and Condiments and Dressings. The categories are the same for all phases of the program, but new "allowable" foods are added for Phase 2 and Phase 3. (There is a column that tells you which foods are allowed in each phase.)

The meal plans are basic guidelines. We tell you the category of foods you are to select from, and you may choose any of the foods in that category *as long as they are approved for your phase level*. For example, if the meal plan says you may choose one serving of a complex carbohydrate, then simply review the list of approved complex carbohydrates and pick whichever one you wish as long as it is approved for your phase.

We also provide a list of "Never" foods. These are items that are off limits during the entire 60-day program. It is truly impossible to list all of the "Never" foods—there are quite literally thousands. It's also impossible to list every single "approved" food, but we have offered plenty of variety so you can enjoy this program and the foods offered. The general guideline is that unless a food is on the "approved" shopping list, you must assume that it is NOT permitted.

> *Model Secret!*
>
> Models, particularly when getting ready for a job, try hard to follow their program very strictly, but if they find that they overindulge one day, then on the next day they will be extra strict and eat more fruits and vegetables and drink extra water to help balance their system.

The program is not all hardship, however. The diet has a built-in reward system—a *Free Day*. IF you follow the diet for 6 days without a slip or a cheat, and IF you have done all of the prescribed workouts, then you have earned one *Free Day* during which you can eat anything you want for a single day. (You've probably done the math, but that means that you could have one *Free Day* every week.) Feel free to eat whatever you like on your *Free Day*, but try to avoid total gluttony! And if you want to skip your *Free Day*, or have a Cheat Meal instead, that will be even better for your ultimate weight loss.

Basic Diet Instructions

- Water is essential. You should drink one 8-ounce glass of water 15 minutes prior to each meal, and you should drink a minimum of 8 glasses of water per day.

- If you do not wish to weigh food servings, the guideline is that one serving is roughly equal to the size of your tightly closed fist, or the amount that will fit into the palm of your hand.

The Venus Summer Shape Up

81

- All methods of cooking are fine except for frying or any method that uses a lot of oil. Anything fried is a "Never."

- When cooking, you may use a small amount of PAM cooking spray or a small amount of Smart Balance butter spread to prevent items from sticking if necessary.

- Eat slowly. Don't "wolf" down your meal. Take your time, eat slowly and enjoy every bite.

Begin by cleaning out your pantry and refrigerator. If others in your home will not be participating in The *Venus Summer Shape Up*, find a way to separate your groceries from any that you won't want to be eating.

Read through how the diet works, make up a grocery list with your favorite healthy foods, and go shopping. Get enough food to last for five or six days worth of meals, and try not to visit the grocery store again until those days are up. Humans are visual creatures. You may think you will just run in to grab some spinach and eggs, but it is very easy to be seduced by the doughnuts and potato chips—especially in the first few weeks. We also suggest you totally avoid fast food restaurants as much as possible, most particularly during the crucial first phase of the program.

Make a copy of the food lists and meal plans. You won't always be at home when you are eating, and you may not always have packed a brown bag full of approved foods. In case you find yourself in unfamiliar food circumstances, make sure you have a copy of the food plan and food choices with you to help you remember the guidelines. And if you are at a restaurant, don't hesitate to make special requests. You'll be surprised at how accommodating most restaurants can be with special requests.

To see sample meals we have created for you be sure to visit Venus.com.

Model Secret!

I try to make good food choices overall, but it's hard during the holidays or when I am traveling. So I just drink a lot of water and do my best to just wait it out till I can get back to my routine and eat healthier foods. Life doesn't always allow you to keep your routines, but you just have to try to balance it out as best you can.

Daily Plans

In each phase, we suggest everyone take three supplements each day:

1. A name brand multivitamin. Most brands are good, but we particularly recommend One-a-Day or Centrum brands.

2. Two 1,000 milligram cholesterol-free Omega 3 supplements. Look for Nordic Naturals or NOW brands.

3. Two 500-600 milligram calcium supplements. Any name brand will be fine.

Each day (in all phases), you can eat 3 meals and 2 snacks:

- Breakfast

- Mid-Morning Snack

- Lunch

- Mid-Day Snack

- Dinner

The Venus Summer Shape Up

BREAKFAST

Select 1 **Protein** and 1 **Complex Carbohydrate**

OR

Select 1 **Protein** and 1 **Fruit**

** In Phase 3, you can add vegetables to this meal **

(for example, if you want to make an omelet from the allowed eggs)

SNACK

Select 1 **Snack** option.

(Note that a low-carb protein shake is the BEST option.)

LUNCH

Select 1 **Protein**, 1 **Fruit**, and 1 **Vegetable**

** In Phase 3 you can add a Complex Carbohydrate to this meal (if desired)
but only IF you are doing all of the Phase 3 workouts.**

SNACK

Select 1 **Snack** option.

(Note that a low-carb protein shake is the BEST option.)

DINNER

Select 1 **Protein** and 1 **Vegetable**

** In Phase 2 you can add 1 fruit to this meal (if desired)
but only IF you are doing all of the Phase 2 workouts **

** In Phase 3 you can add 1 dessert to this meal (if desired)
but only IF you are doing all of the Phase 3 workouts.**

APPROVED FOODS

Protein

Phases Meats | | Amounts

Phases	Meats	Amounts
1, 2, 3	Skinless Chicken Breast	3 oz
1, 2, 3	Skinless Turkey Breast	3 oz
1, 2, 3	Lean Ground Beef (95% fat free)	3 oz
1, 2, 3	Lean Ground Turkey Breast	3 oz
1, 2, 3	Lean Steak	3 oz
1, 2, 3	Lean Pork	3 oz
1, 2, 3	Buffalo	3 oz

Fish & Seafood

Phases		Amounts
1, 2, 3	Salmon	4 oz
1, 2, 3	White Tuna (fresh or canned in water)	4 oz
1, 2, 3	Shellfish (all)	4 oz
1, 2, 3	Clams - canned in water	4 oz
1, 2, 3	Lobster - Steamed	4 oz
1, 2, 3	Shrimp - Steamed	4 oz
1, 2, 3	Blue Crab - Canned	4 oz
1, 2, 3	Tilapia	4 oz
1, 2, 3	Mahi	4 oz
1, 2, 3	Grouper	4 oz
1, 2, 3	Flounder	4 oz

Dairy

Phases		Amounts
1, 2, 3	Eggs (whole)	2 eggs
1, 2, 3	Egg Whites or Egg Substitute	3 egg equiv.
1, 2, 3	Low Fat Cottage Cheese	1 cup
1, 2, 3	Tofu	1/2 cup

Complex Carbohydrates

Phases	Carbs	Amounts
1, 2, 3	Whole Wheat Bread	1 slice
1, 2, 3	Whole Wheat Pasta	1 cup
1, 2, 3	Whole Oats	1/2 cup
2, 3	Grits	1/2 cup
2, 3	Brown Rice	1/2 cup
3	Potato	1 medium
3	Sweet Potato	1 medium
3	Whole Wheat Bagel	1/4 bagel

Fruits

Phases	Fruits	Amounts
1, 2, 3	Apple	1 medium
1, 2, 3	Banana	1 medium
1, 2, 3	Berries	1 cup
1, 2, 3	Cantaloupe	1 cup
1, 2, 3	Grapes	1 cup
1, 2, 3	Grapefruit	1/2 medium
1, 2, 3	Lemon or Lime	unlimited
1, 2, 3	Orange	1 medium
1, 2, 3	Pear	1 medium
1, 2, 3	Strawberries	1 cup

Vegetables*

Phases	Vegetables	Amounts
1, 2, 3	Any Green Vegetable	1 cup
1, 2, 3	Beans (any)	1/2 cup
1, 2, 3	Cabbage	unlimited
1, 2, 3	Carrots	1/2 cup
1, 2, 3	Cauliflower	1 cup
1, 2, 3	Celery	unlimited
1, 2, 3	Cucumber	unlimited
1, 2, 3	Lettuce (any variety)	unlimited
1, 2, 3	Mushrooms (raw)	1 cup
1, 2, 3	Onions	unlimited
1, 2, 3	Peas	1 cup
1, 2, 3	Tomatoes	1 cup
1, 2, 3	Zucchini	unlimited

* When you have a vegetable option you can combine any of these to make a salad.

Beverages

Phases	Drink	Amounts
1, 2, 3	Water	8 glasses/day (min)
1, 2, 3	Black Coffee	unlimited
1, 2, 3	Unsweetened Black or Green Tea	unlimited
2, 3	Skim Milk	2 cups/day limit
2, 3	Soy Milk	2 cups/day limit
3	Alcohol	1 drink/day limit
3	Diet Soda	12 oz/day limit
3	Sugar-free water drinks*	unlimited

* Note: sugar-free water drinks are usually sweet, and we want to break the addiction to sweet things in phases 1 and 2.

Snacks

Phases	Snack	Amounts
1, 2, 3	Protein Shake (25 carb max) mixed w/water	
2, 3	Protein Shake (25 carb max) mixed w/water, milk, or soy milk	
Best Protein Shake choices:	EAS 100% Whey Protein	
	Designer Whey	
1, 2, 3	Protein Bar (25 carb max)	1 bar
Best Protein Bar choices:	1.5-oz Detour bars	
	Pure Protein bars	
	Atkins Bars	
	South Beach High Protein Cereal Bars	
1, 2, 3	Almonds	1 ounce
1, 2, 3	Pumpkin Seeds	1 cup
1, 2, 3	Sunflower Seeds	1/4 cup
1, 2, 3	Pistachio Nuts	1 ounce
1, 2, 3	Walnuts	1 ounce
1, 2, 3	Low-fat, no-sugar Peanut Butter	1 tablespoon
1, 2, 3	Sugar-free gum	unlimited
1, 2, 3	Cheese (shredded), low-fat or no-fat	1/2 cup
1, 2, 3	Low-fat Cottage Cheese	1 cup
2, 3	Yogurt, no-fat or low fat	6 ounces

Desserts

Phases	Dessert	Amounts
3	Sugar-free gelatin dessert	1 serving
3	Sugar-free Pudding	1 serving

Dressings and Condiments

Phases	Dressings/Condiments	Amounts
1, 2, 3	Mustard	unlimited
1, 2, 3	Low-fat Mayo	1 tablespoon
1, 2, 3	Low-fat Salad Dressing (any)	2 tablespoons/salad
1, 2, 3	Smart Balance butter spread	1 teaspoon/day
1, 2, 3	Vinaigrette	4 tablespoons
1, 2, 3	Salad dressing spritzers	unlimited
1, 2, 3	Zero Calorie Butter spray	unlimited
3	Non-fat Cream Cheese	1 tablesp. twice/week

NEVER!

White Bread	None of any sort
White Rice	None of any sort
Regular Soda	None of any sort
Sweet Tea	None of any sort
Sugar	None of any sort
Fried Foods	None of any sort
Cold Breakfast cereals	None are acceptable
Bagels	Except as noted
Most Salad Dressings	Except as noted
** High Fructose Corn Syrup	None of any sort
** Trans Fats	None of any sort

**You will need to check ingredient lists for these ingredients

Chapter 9:
Move Like a Model—
3 Phases of Exercise

This is the most exciting part of The *Venus Summer Shape Up*, the part that is going to fire up your metabolism, tighten your thighs, boost your butt, and give you the kind of abs that will make you want to show them off!

In all probability, you are currently getting very little exercise. One survey found that only 25% of us engage in any sort of regular physical activity. When did exercise get to be such a chore? When we were kids, we loved moving. Without even thinking about it we were out running and jumping and playing—and we loved it! There is joy in the freedom that comes from being strong enough to run around the block, ride a bike to the park, or go swimming all afternoon. Children feel muscle happiness with every leap or spin. Where did it go?

It's there, inside your own muscles, just waiting to be released! But you'll never know how good you can feel until you bring back that joy of movement into your life. Obviously, we would like everyone to eat well and exercise for the rest of their lives. But for right now, we're willing to settle for the next 60 days. Commit yourself to our program for just 60 days, and at the end of those 60 days, if you don't enjoy feeling slimmer and more energetic, by all means feel free to stop. But I'm willing to bet that you won't want to quit. I predict that you'll find your passion for fitness somewhere around week 4 and then you'll be enthused about your workouts. Fitness starts in the mind. If you believe that you are capable of overcoming any obstacle, then you are already most of the way there. The mental aspect is about 75% of the process. If you can visualize your goal, you can achieve it. Believe in yourself—you are more powerful than you've given yourself credit for!

Where to Start

Each phase of The *Venus Summer Shape Up* program lasts 20 days. We recommend that everyone start with Phase One—the Beginner level. ***It will challenge you!*** Don't jump ahead to the next level unless you've already been exercising on a consistent basis, even if the exercises begin to feel easy. Each stage of our program is designed to prepare your body for the next stage. Your body needs time to adapt to new routines before we start adding additional exercises to the program. In addition, if you jump ahead before your body adapts, you will be more prone to injury and that will set you back.

This program was developed by Skip Sylvester, the *Venus* fitness trainer, a power lifting and bodybuilding champion who has been helping people shape their bodies for more than 20 years. He works with professional athletes, CEOs, celebrities, and people just like you—women who want to be slimmer, stronger, and physically younger. On Skip's program, you'll cover both major areas of fitness training—aerobic exercise and strength training—with options for doing the exercises at home <u>OR</u> at a gym. The scope of the program may seem like a lot at times, but don't worry about rushing it. We promise you'll be able to do it all if you take it one step at a time.

> *Model Secret!*
>
> My motto is "No Negativity"! Negativity breeds more negativity, and soon you get caught in a downward spiral. Think positive all the time. Eventually you'll rework your psyche and become more self-confident and self-assured.

Basic Exercise Instructions

• Obligatory note of caution: These exercises are designed for healthy people who have received approval from their doctor to engage in physical exercise. You should not attempt these exercises unless your personal physician has told you that you can engage in vigorous physical exercise.

• When you do aerobic exercise in the beginning phase, you will aim for an intensity that you can maintain for the entire time required. For most people, that means walking, jogging, biking, swimming, rollerblading, etc. at a pace that will have you breathing heavily, but still be able to hold a normal conversation. If you are so out of breath that you can't talk in a normal conversational tone, then you're pushing too hard in the beginning phase. You'll work harder in phase two, and in the third phase you'll do some "interval training," which means that during parts of that workout, you might not be able to hold a conversation, but that's for later…. After a few days, you'll be able to judge your capabilities more easily.

• Resistance or Strength training exercises can be done at a **gym** using the equipment there **OR** at **home** with just a couple of dumbbells. While the gym workout is preferred, either will give you a good workout. The exercises below are grouped by location.

> **Gym Phase One** begins on page 102, and continues through Gym Phase Three.

> **Home Phase One** begins on page 138, and continues through Home Phase Three.

> **It is okay to mix it up** with gym and home exercises. For each level, the exercises are grouped in such a way that you can do the exercises at the gym one day and then do the corresponding home version of that phase for the next workout if you can't get back to the gym.

- If using the machines at the gym is a new experience for you, ask one of the trainers there to give you tips on how to adjust the equipment for your height and exercise level. Note that the type and brand of machines vary from gym to gym. The machines at your gym may not EXACTLY match the machines we show in our examples. If this is the case, ask for help from the trainers at your gym. They will have comparable equipment that will allow you to complete this workout.

- The resistance exercises must be done in the exact order given to maximize the effectiveness of the program.

- Each exercise has a specific form and we provide photographs of *Venus* model Jessiqa performing the exercise, as well as a description of how to do the exercise properly. If you are not used to working with machines or dumbbells, these exercises may feel awkward at first. Be patient—it will soon feel as natural as brushing your hair.

- Resistance exercises have their own vocabulary.

> *Repetitions (or Reps):* Reps refer to the number of times each individual exercise needs to be performed, one right after the other. If you are doing sit-ups, for example, each sit-up counts as one "rep." Do 25 sit-ups, one right after the next, and that is "25 reps." Each exercise in this program needs to be repeated at least 10 times in a row. That means 10 reps. The specific number of reps you do will vary depending on your level and the particular exercise. Each rep is done one right after the other, without resting in between.

> **Set:** A group of reps is called a set. After you finish 10 reps, for example, that group of 10 would be one set of reps for that exercise. After each set you should rest for 30-60 seconds.

Then, you'll begin another set. In this program, you'll need to do two or more sets of each exercise. For example, if the exercise calls for three sets of 10 reps, you'll do a total of 30 reps. You will do one set of 10 reps, rest for 30-60 seconds, do a second set of 10 reps, rest for 30-60 seconds and then do your final set of 10 reps. That's three total sets for 30 total reps. After you complete all of the sets for a given exercise, move on to the next exercise.

Here's What You Need to Begin

- **Access to a gym OR a set of dumbbells from 2½ to 8 pounds (two of each weight).** You can get dumbbells in weights of 2½ pounds, 3 pounds, 4 pounds, 5 pounds and 8 pounds.

- **Comfortable work-out clothes.** Choose clothing that allows you to move freely without pulling, pinching, bunching, or riding up.

- **Sneakers.** These should provide good support to help keep you balanced. A good pair of cross-trainers will serve double duty—in the gym for weight training, and on the street or treadmill for aerobic exercise.

- **Towel.** To wipe any sweat off of the gym machines.

- **Watch or clock.** In order to time your rests between sets, you'll need to have access to a clock or watch with a second hand. All gyms should have at least one large clock, so you probably won't need to bring one along.

- **Water.** Drink plenty of water before and after your aerobic workouts. We suggest you bring a water bottle with you for your strength training workouts so that you can sip water between sets.

- **Music Helps.** When I cycle, run, or work out, I always use my iPod to listen to upbeat music that helps keep me moving and motivated.

Model Secret!

When I do strength training, I like to wear clothes that are more form-fitting (as opposed to baggy sweatpants and sweatshirt). That way, I can more easily see the way my muscles are moving and I can better focus on the correct form.

BONUS EXERCISES...

Once you have completed Phase Three, which has the most advanced exercises, we know you'll be hungry for something more. That's why we've included special bonus exercises using a Swiss ball. These exercises can be tricky and quite difficult, so please do not attempt them unless you feel ready to move on to the next level. Descriptions of the Swiss Ball exercises begin on page 170.

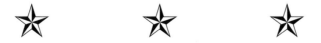

Are you ready? Here we go!

Schedule for all phases:

Aerobics: 5 to 7 days per week, 30 minutes per day.

Strength: 3 days per week, with at least 1 day of rest between workouts. The strength or resistance exercises should take about 30 minutes for Phase One, 40 minutes for Phase Two, and 50 minutes for Phase Three.

Sample Schedule:

Monday: 30 minutes of aerobic exercise in the morning.
Strength Training in the late afternoon prior to dinner.

Tuesday: 30 minutes of aerobic exercise in the morning.

Wednesday: 30 minutes of aerobic exercise in the morning.
Strength Training in the late afternoon prior to dinner.

Thursday: 30 minutes of aerobic exercise in the morning

Friday: 30 minutes of aerobic exercise in the morning.
Strength Training in the late afternoon prior to dinner.

Saturday: 30 minutes of aerobic exercise in the morning.

Sunday: OFF

Aerobic Training

Any kind of aerobic exercise you enjoy will work just fine. The only real guidelines are that your body must be moving, and it must make you breathe a little heavily. Walking is a terrific aerobic exercise, as long as you walk fast enough to become slightly winded. A gentle stroll just won't do it.

Walking and jogging are the most common and easiest of the aerobic exercises since they require nothing other than good footwear and access to safe streets or a treadmill. Other options are to bike, hike, swim, row, do guided aerobics in a class or with a DVD, take a spinning class, use an elliptical trainer or stair climber ... anything that gets you breathing hard and increases your heart rate will do the job.

When it comes to aerobics, the more you do, the more successful you will be and the quicker your body will change! You can mix it up if you like: bike one day, jog the next, and then do an aerobics class. You can do aerobics every day, or even twice a day if you wish. There's almost no such thing as too much when it comes to aerobic exercise. Our 30 minute suggestion is the minimum.

AEROBICS—Moving through the Phases

Although the specifics will change with the types of exercises you choose, the following descriptions use walking and jogging as examples. The goal is to push yourself a little harder with each level.

Measure your effort on a personal 1-to-10 scale, where 1 is sitting in a recliner doing nothing but tapping your foot, and 10 is MAXIMUM effort. If you hit 10, you'll be saying to yourself that you can't keep this up...can't breathe...can't talk. As you move from phase to phase, you'll want to challenge yourself more, but you'll also notice that your personal 1-to-10 scale will change as your body becomes stronger. (Guidelines are listed for each phase on the next page.)

All aerobic workouts should be 30 minutes minimum, 5 days per week minimum.

AEROBIC PHASE ONE: Start walking briskly outside or on a treadmill. Periodically break into a jog, even if it's only for 10 to 15 seconds. Then resume walking. Repeat this pattern—walk/jog...walk/jog...walk/jog. Keep your level of effort at about a 6 on that 1 to 10 scale. At this level, you'll be breathing hard and steady, but you'll still be able to carry on a normal conversation with a partner. If you choose to wear a heart rate monitor, that's even better. You'll want to keep your pulse between 60% and 70% of your maximum heart rate for the whole 30 minutes. You can calculate your approximate maximum heart rate by deducting your age from 220. Thus, if you are 40, your approximate maximum heart rate is 180. So at this phase you would strive to keep your heart rate between 108 (which is 60% of 180, calculated by multiplying 0.6 x 180) and 126 (which is 70% of 180, calculated by multiplying 0.7 x 180).

You will perform PHASE ONE for 20 days and then move on to PHASE TWO.

AEROBIC PHASE TWO: At this intermediate level, your exertion should be greater. Strive for a 7 or 8 on your personal effort level. You should be breathing harder and faster, and be able to speak in short sentences but not carry on a normal conversation. If you choose to wear a heart rate monitor, keep your pulse between 70% and 80% of your max heart rate for the whole 30 minutes. Depending on your fitness level, this will probably still be a walk/jog combo, but with more jogging and less walking.

You will perform PHASE TWO for 20 days and then move on to PHASE THREE.

AEROBIC PHASE THREE: At the advanced level, you'll start to do true interval training. This is where you'll really begin to push it. Begin by jogging slowly and steadily to warm up, but then push it! Jog hard and fast, pushing your exertion to about a 9 on your personal effort scale. Then slow down to a slow jog or walk until you get back to a 7. Then crank it up again, going back up to a 9. Use this interval technique throughout the whole workout. If you choose to wear a heart rate monitor, begin slowly to warm up and then push it to get your pulse to about 85% - 90% of your max heart rate, and then slow down until your pulse slows back down to 70%-75%, then repeat the process. Do this "interval" training for the whole 30 minutes of your aerobic workout.

Strength Training—at the Gym

The following pages contain the gym-based strength training program for all phases of The *Venus Summer Shape Up*.
(The Home program begins on page 138)

Work through each exercise in the order listed for the phase you are in. Because all gyms and all machines are slightly different, it is impossible to assign a specific weight amount for each exercise. When in doubt, start light. Most exercises require you to do 10-12 reps. During your first set, you should be able to complete 12 reps. During your second and third sets, you should be challenged to complete the last 2 or 3 reps. If you can't complete at least 10 reps in your first set, lower the weight. If you can do 12 reps in all three sets without significant effort, move to a higher weight. Always endeavor to add weight as you go from workout to workout, but stick with 10 reps as your minimum.

Be the best you can be, each and every day!

Workout Tips

- Proper form is crucial. Each rep should be done in a slow and controlled manner. If you aren't using proper form or you are swinging the weights the weight is too heavy. Select a lighter weight.

- If you can do the maximum number of reps listed for all of the required sets you should move to a heavier weight at the next workout.

- Bring a small notebook to keep track of your weights and reps. After 45 days go back and review your first workouts. Look at how much progress you've made! You're stronger - it's working!

- For each rep there is a "work phase" where you are pushing or pulling to move the weight and a "release phase" where you are returning the weight to the starting position. Generally you should do the "work phase" to the count of 2 as you exhale and do the "release phase" slowly, to the count of 4, as you inhale.

- Rest 30-60 seconds between sets.

- Soreness in your muscles the first week or so is to be expected. Stick with it! The soreness will go away.

Phase One: Wake-Up Call!

The following pages contain the gym version of the strength training program for all phases of the Venus Summer Shape Up Program.

When you begin the program, start light. Most exercises require you to complete 10-12 reps. During your first set, you should be able to complete 12 reps. During your second and third sets, it should be a challenge for you to complete the last 2 or 3 reps. If you can't complete at least 10 reps in your first set, lower the weight. If you can do 12 reps with good form in all three sets, move to a higher weight during your next workout.

Don't take "no" for an answer—you're worth the extra effort!

- ## Medium-grip barbell bench press
  ## 3 Sets   10-12 Reps

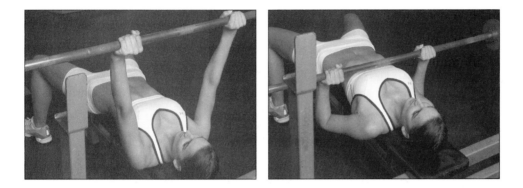

STEPS

1. Lie on your back on the bench. Grip the bar with your hands positioned just outside your shoulder width.

2. Slowly lower the weight to about the level of your breasts.

3. Press the weight back up, then repeat.

KEEP IN MIND

- Your back and head should remain motionless.

- It is also important to expand your rib cage by inhaling deeply when you lower the bar to your chest. Exhale as you push the bar back up.

Wide-grip front pull-down machine
3 Sets   10-12 Reps

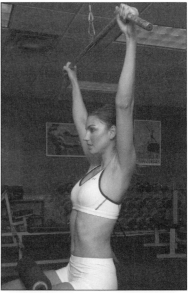

STEPS

1. Sit down and hold the bar with both hands (outside your shoulder width).

2. Pull the bar down and try to touch your upper chest, while squeezing your shoulder blades together.

3. Slowly release, and guide the bar back up to the starting position so that your arms are extended fully. Repeat.

KEEP IN MIND

- You may lean back slightly.

- Exaggerate pushing your chest out, while simultaneously squeezing your shoulder blades together.

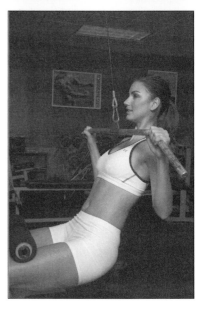

• Military press
3 Sets   10-12 Reps

STEPS

1. Stand with feet shoulder width apart and hold the dumbbells at shoulder level, palms facing forward.

2. Press the weight up above your head until your arms are fully extended.

3. Slowly lower the weight to the starting position, and repeat.

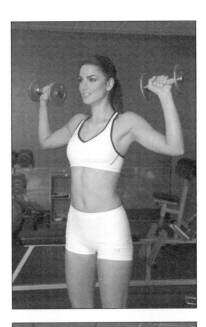

KEEP IN MIND

• Do your reps with very slow, very controlled movements to reduce the chance of injury.

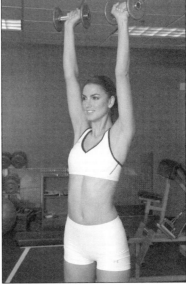

- ## Close-grip easy curl bar
  ## 3 Sets   10-12 Reps

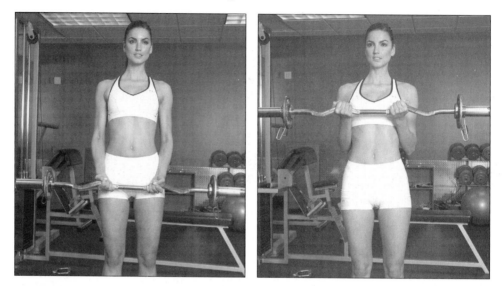

STEPS

1. From a standing position, hold the bar with both hands palm up, with a narrow grip.

2. Keeping your elbows by your side, raise the bar up, and squeeze your biceps at the top of the motion.

3. Lower the bar slowly all the way down to your starting position, and repeat.

KEEP IN MIND

- Your elbows should remain at your sides at all times. This will keep the tension on your bicep muscles instead of your shoulders.

- Do not "rock" your upper body to swing the weight up. Your upper body should remain motionless so your biceps do all the work.

- ## Tricep press down machine, overhand
  ## 3 Sets   10-12 Reps

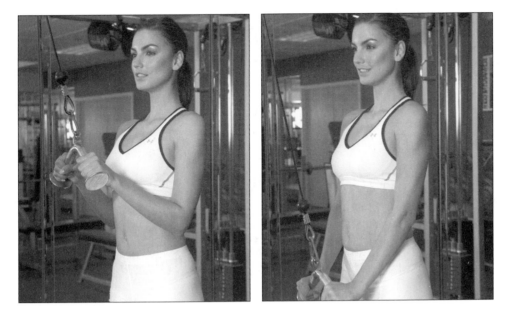

STEPS

1. Hold the bar with a close grip, palms facing the floor. Concentrate on keeping your elbows positioned at your sides.

2. Bring the weight down slowly by straightening your arms, and then bring them back up to the starting position. Repeat.

KEEP IN MIND

- Your form is everything on this exercise. Keep your elbows tight against your sides, and use very slow movements.

• Lying hamstring curl
3 Sets   10-12 Reps

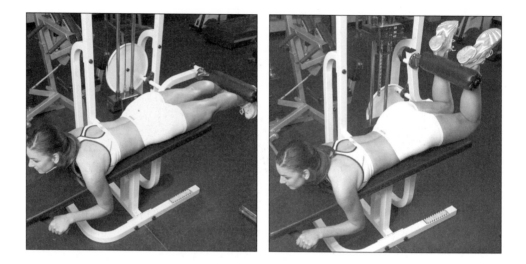

STEPS

1. Lie face down on the machine and place your heels under the foot pad.

2. Curl your legs until the pad touches your upper legs.

3. Slowly let the pad down to the starting position, and repeat.

KEEP IN MIND

• Don't jerk or pull with your lower back. This can result in a muscle strain.

- ## Thigh extension
  ### 3 Sets   10-12 Reps

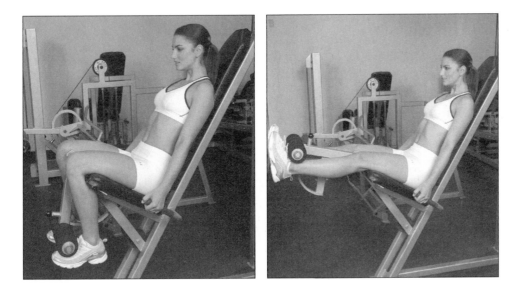

STEPS

1. Sit down on the machine and hook your feet under the foot pads.

2. Extend your legs straight out until they are almost fully extended.

3. Slowly bring the weight back down to the starting position, and repeat.

KEEP IN MIND

- Be careful not to lock your knees when your legs are extended. This puts undue stress on your knees.

• Standing calf machine
3 Sets   25-30 Reps

STEPS

1. Stand on the machine on the balls of your feet.

2. Lower your heels as far as possible to create a full stretch.

3. Then, push up as far as you can on your tip toes.

4. Then, lower slowly and repeat.

KEEP IN MIND

• Machines may vary. If your gym's machine is significantly different from the one described here, ask a trainer for instructions.

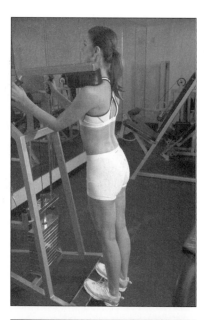

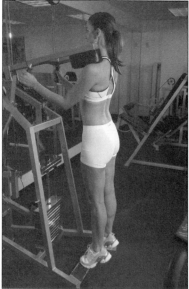

- ## Crunches
  ## 3 Sets   10-20 Reps

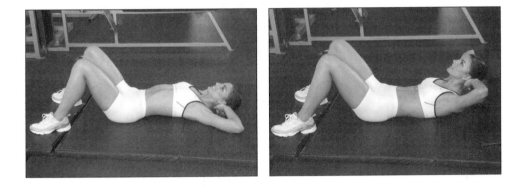

STEPS

1. Lie on your back, with your knees bent and your feet on the floor. Place your hands behind your head or across your chest.

2. Lift your torso towards the ceiling. Breathe out on the upward movement.

3. Lower your torso, and repeat.

KEEP IN MIND

- You should feel constant tension in your abs, not your neck or back.

Phase Two: Transformation

*In Phase Two, you will need to do
ALL exercises listed for Phase 1,
PLUS one or two additional exercises
per muscle group. Do the exercises
in the order listed. (Photographs and
descriptions are only provided for the exercises
that are new additions to this phase.)*

- ## Medium-grip barbell bench press

(Gym - Phase One)

2 Sets   10-12 Reps

- ## Inner-pec press
2 Sets   10-12 Reps

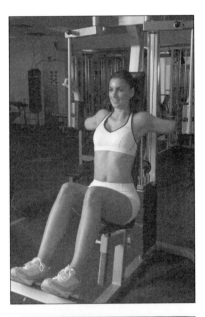

STEPS

1. Sit down at the pec deck machine. Hold the handles, and place your elbows against the pads. Push your chest out and up. Your upper back will be touching the pad.

2. Contract your pectoral (chest) muscles, and bring the two arm pads together in front of you.

3. Slowly open your arms as far as you comfortably can, then repeat.

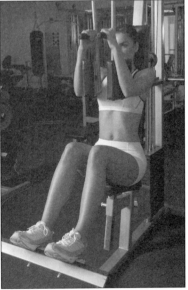

KEEP IN MIND

- Only stretch as far as you can comfortably. Stretching too far back can cause undue stress on your shoulders.

113

- ## Wide-grip front pull-down *(Gym - Phase One)*
  ## 2 Sets   10-12 Reps

- ## Narrow-grip seated row
  ## 2 Sets   10-12 Reps

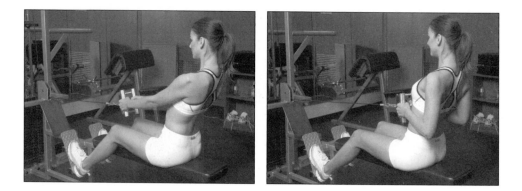

STEPS

1. Sit down and grasp the handle with a close grip.

2. Pull the handle into your upper stomach, just below your chest. Push your chest out and squeeze your shoulder blades together.

3. Release slowly for a full stretch, and repeat.

KEEP IN MIND

- Do not "round" your lower back during the stretch portion of the movement. This can cause stress on the lower back muscles.

- **Military Press** *(Gym - Phase One)*
  ## 2 Sets   10-12 Reps

- **Side laterals**
  ## 2 Sets   10-12 Reps

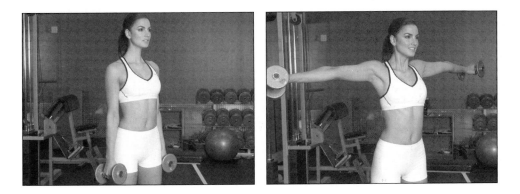

STEPS

1. Stand and hold the dumbbells at your sides, with your palms facing inward.

2. Raise your arms out to your sides, lifting to a parallel position with your shoulders.

3. Lower the weight slowly to the starting position. Repeat.

KEEP IN MIND

- There should be a slight bend in your elbows. Only raise the dumb bells to a parallel position.

- ## Close-grip easy curl bar *(Gym - Phase One)*
  ## 2 Sets   10-12 Reps

- ## Hammer curl
  ## 2 Sets   10-12 Reps

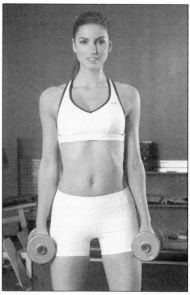

STEPS

1. Stand and hold the dumbbells by your sides, with your palms facing inward.

2. Keeping your elbows positioned by your sides, raise the dumbbells up as far as possible toward your shoulders.

3. Slowly lower the dumbbells to the starting position, and repeat.

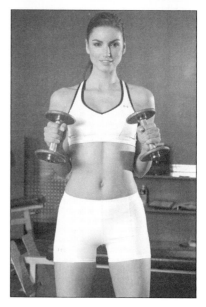

KEEP IN MIND

- Your hand position is very important on this exercise. Keep palms in to maintain the intensity on the right muscles.

- ## Tricep press down overhand *(Gym - Phase One)*
  ## 2 Sets   10-12 Reps

- ## Tricep press down underhand
  ## 2 Sets   10-12 Reps

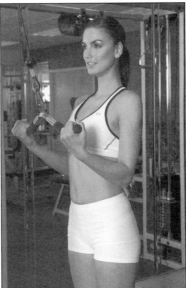

STEPS

1. Stand, and grasp the bar with a close grip, with your palms facing the ceiling.

2. With your elbows at your sides, bring the weight down slowly.

3. Return to the starting position. Repeat.

KEEP IN MIND

- Concentrate on keeping your elbows positioned at your sides.

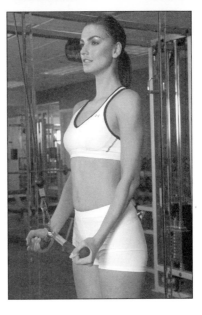

117

- # Lying hamstring curl *(Gym - Phase One)*
  ## 2 Sets   10-12 Reps

- # Thigh extension
  (Gym - Phase One)
  ## 2 Sets   10-12 Reps

- # Squat **OR** Leg press
  ## 2 Sets   10-12 Reps

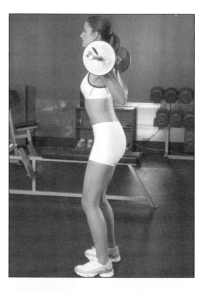

STEPS: SQUAT

1. Position the bar on your upper back (across your shoulders), with your feet shoulder-width apart.

2. Keeping your back straight and your feet flat on the floor, lower your body to a squatting position.

3. Do not squat so deep that you allow your butt to dip below the level of your knees.

4. Push up to the starting position. Repeat.

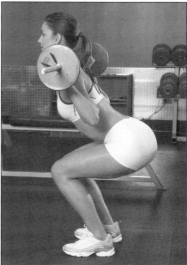

KEEP IN MIND

- Keep your back straight, as shown in photo. Do not allow your back to "round" forward as this could strain your lower back.

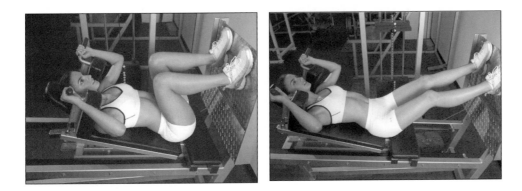

STEPS: LEG PRESS

1. Place your feet on the plate, shoulder-width apart.

2. Lower the weight until your hips and lower legs are at a 90° angle.

3. Push up to the starting position. Repeat.

KEEP IN MIND

• Keep your back flat on the padded surface.

- ## Walking lunges
  ## 2 Sets   10-12 Reps

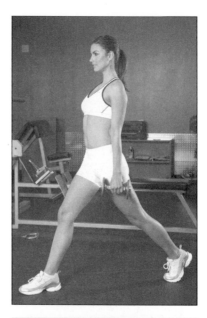

STEPS

1. Stand and hold the dumbbells by your sides.

2. Take a long stride forward and lower your rear knee until it is just off the floor.

3. Push yourself up, step forward with the other leg, and repeat the movement.

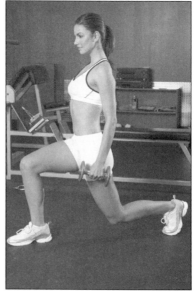

KEEP IN MIND

- Each step counts as one rep.

- For the first few times, start with no weight in your hands.

- Don't allow your forward knee to extend over your front foot on any repetition.

● Standing calf machine
4 Sets   25 Reps

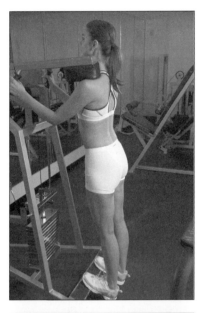

Note: For Phase Two we've added one extra set.

STEPS

1. Stand on the machine on the balls of your feet.

2. Lower your heels as far as possible to create a full stretch.

3. Then, push up as far as you can on your tip toes.

4. Then, lower slowly and repeat.

KEEP IN MIND

- Machines may vary. If your gym's machine is significantly different from the one described here, ask a trainer for instructions.

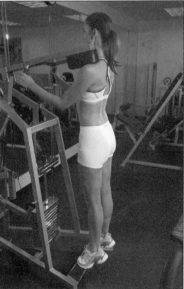

121

- ## Crunches *(Gym - Phase One)*
  ### 3 Sets   10-20 Reps

- ## Leg lifts
  ### 3 Sets   10-20 Reps

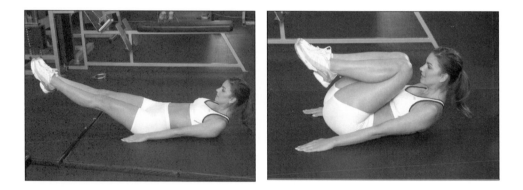

STEPS

1. Lie on your back and place your arms down at your sides with your palms down.

2. Lift your legs 6 inches off of the ground, then bend your knees and pull your legs inward towards your chest. (Breathe out when you are pulling your legs inward.)

3. Extend your legs back out to the starting position, and repeat.

KEEP IN MIND

- You should only feel stress on your abdominals, not your neck or back.

Phase Three: Energizing

**For the GYM workout, do ALL exercises listed
for Phase One and Phase Two, but only two
sets, PLUS the one or two additional
exercises shown here, per muscle group.
Do the exercises in the order listed.
(Photographs and descriptions are only
provided for the exercises that are new
additions to this phase.)**

- ## Medium-grip barbell bench press *(Gym - Phase One)*
  ## 2 Sets   10-12 Reps

- ## Inner-pec press *(Gym - Phase Two)*
  ## 2 Sets   10-12 Reps

- ## Palms-in dumbbell press
  ## 2 Sets   10-12 Reps

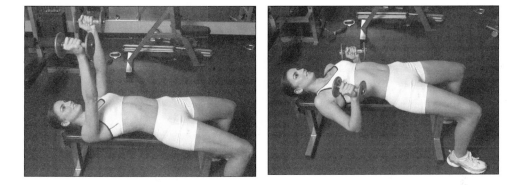

STEPS

1. While lying on a flat or incline bench, hold the dumbbells in your hands, palms facing in, arms extended straight out from your body.

2. Slowly lower the dumbbells down beside your chest.

3. Press the dumbbells back up to the starting position. Repeat.

KEEP IN MIND

- Hand position is very important on this exercise to insure the stress is on your chest and not your shoulders.

125

- ## Wide-grip front pull-down *(Gym - Phase One)*
  ## 2 Sets   10-12 Reps

- ## Narrow-grip seated row *(Gym - Phase Two)*
  ## 2 Sets   10-12 Reps

- ## Underhand grip pull-down **OR** Assisted pull-up
  ## 2 Sets   10-12 Reps

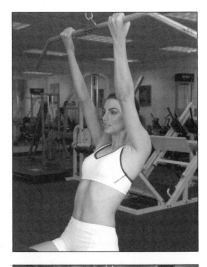

STEPS: UNDERHAND GRIP PULL-DOWN

1. Sit down and hold the bar with a close grip, your palms facing towards you.

2. Pull the bar down to your upper chest, and squeeze your shoulder blades together.

3. Slowly return the bar to the starting position, and repeat.

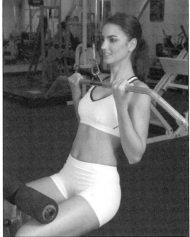

STEPS: ASSISTED PULL-UP:

1. Grab the bar with an overhand grip, palms facing away from you.

2. Pull your torso up towards the ceiling. Push your chest upward and squeeze your shoulder blades together.

3. Lower yourself slowly. Repeat.

KEEP IN MIND

- This exercise is one of the hardest because it recruits more of your upper body muscles than most any other exercise.

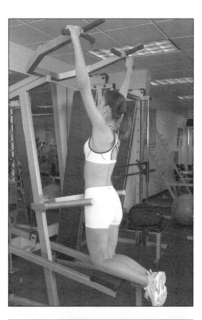

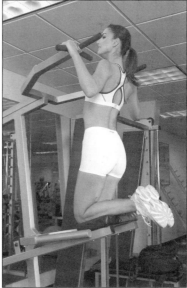

- **Military Press** *(Gym - Phase One)*
  ## 2 Sets   10-12 Reps

- **Side laterals** *(Gym - Phase Two)*
  ## 2 Sets   10-12 Reps

- **Rear delt raise**
  ## 2 Sets   10-12 Reps

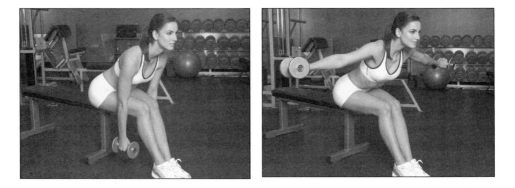

STEPS

1. Sit on the end of the bench, and bend your torso over your knees. Hold the dumbbells with your palms facing inward.

2. Start with the dumbbells under your knees, and then raise them out to your sides. It is important to stay bent over.

3. Lower the dumbbells slowly to the starting position. Repeat.

KEEP IN MIND

- The stress is on your rear delts, not on your lower back.

- ## Close-grip easy curl bar *(Gym - Phase One)*
  ## 2 Sets   10-12 Reps

- ## Hammer curl
  (Gym - Phase Two)
  ## 2 Sets   10-12 Reps

- ## Cable curls
  ## 2 Sets   10-12 Reps

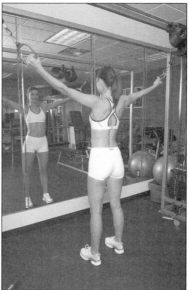

STEPS

1. Stand with a cable handle in each hand, arms extended.

2. Contract your biceps, pulling your hands toward your ears.

3. Squeeze your biceps, then release all the way to the starting position. Repeat.

KEEP IN MIND

- Your elbows should be slightly higher than your shoulders. This will keep the emphasis on your biceps.

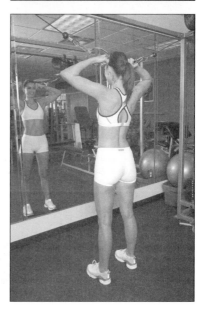

129

- **Tricep press down overhand** *(Gym - Phase One)*
  2 Sets   10-12 Reps

- **Tricep press down underhand** *(Gym - Phase Two)*
  2 Sets   10-12 Reps

- **Easy curl bar extension lying down**
  2 Sets   10-12 Reps

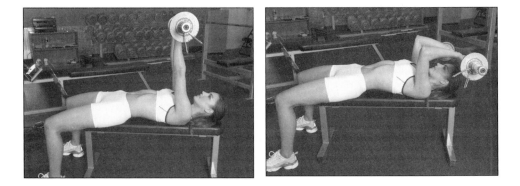

STEPS

1. Lie on your back, and hold the easy-curl bar above your head, palms facing away from you.

2. Bend at the elbows, and lower the bar to a position just behind your forehead. Keep your elbows pulled inward, toward your chest.

3. Press the bar back up to the starting position. Repeat.

KEEP IN MIND

- Be careful when lowering the bar near your head.

- Lying hamstring curl *(Gym - Phase One)*
  2 Sets   10-12 Reps

- Thigh extension *(Gym - Phase One)*
  2 Sets   10-12 Reps

- Squat OR Leg Press *(Gym - Phase Two)*
  2 Sets   10-12 Reps

- Walking lunges *(Gym - Phase Two)*
  2 Sets   10-12 Reps

- ## Straight leg dead lifts **OR**
  ## Step-ups on box
  ## 2 Sets   10-12 Reps

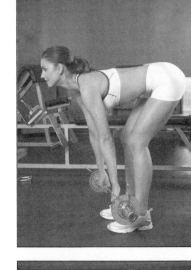

STEPS

1. Stand with your feet shoulder-width apart and your knees slightly bent. Hold the bar close to your body at the level of your thighs, palms facing in toward your legs.

2. Keeping your back flat and your knees slightly bent, lower the bar as far as possible.

3. Straighten back up, and repeat.

KEEP IN MIND

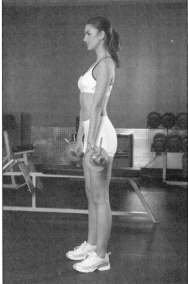

- Keep the bar close to your legs, not dangling out away from your body.

- Remember to keep your back flat, not rounded. This will keep the emphasis on your hamstrings and butt without stressing your lower back.

• Step-ups on box
2 Sets   10-12 Reps

STEPS

Prep: You will need a box, step, or chair that is at least 15" to 18" in height.

1. Stand facing the box, step, or chair.

2. Step up with your right leg first, and follow with your left.

3. Then, step down with your left leg first.

4. Repeat until all 10-12 reps are complete on your right leg. Then repeat your 10-12 reps, leading with your left leg.

KEEP IN MIND

• Keep your torso upright, do not lean forward. This will keep the emphasis on your glutes and hamstrings.

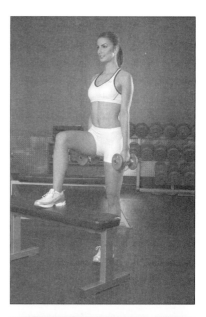

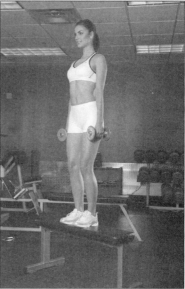

- ## Standing calf machine *(Gym - Phase One)*
  ## 3 Sets   25 Reps

- ## Toe raises
  ## 3 Sets   10-12 Reps

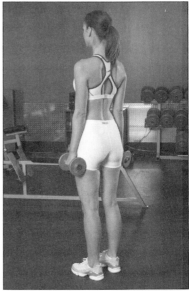

STEPS

1. Stand with your dumbbells at your side.

2. Lift your heels until you are on the tip of your toes.

3. Lower back down to the floor. Repeat.

KEEP IN MIND

- Pause at the top of this movement to flex your calf muscles.

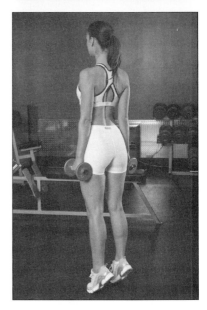

- **Crunches** *(Gym - Phase One)*
  2 Sets   10-20 Reps

- **Leg lifts** *(Gym - Phase Two)*
  2 Sets   10-20 Reps

- ## Core ball leg lift and Crunch
  ## 2 Sets   10-20 Reps

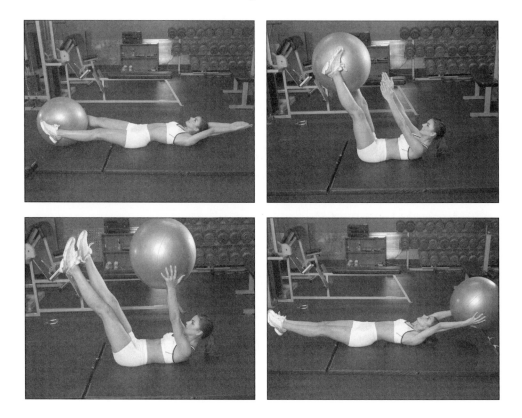

STEPS

1. Lie on your back with the core ball between your knees and ankles.

2. Lift your legs and torso simultaneously, and grab the ball with your hands.

3. Lower your torso and legs to the starting position, with the ball over your head.

4. Raise your torso and legs back up, and place the ball back between your knees and ankles.

5. Return to the starting position, and repeat.

KEEP IN MIND

• This is an advanced exercise--do your repetitions slowly and with great control.

Phase One: Strength Training

The following pages contain the home-based strength training program for all phases of the Venus Summer Shape Up. (The Gym program begins on page 102.)

Work through each exercise in the order listed for the phase you are in. For exercises that require dumbbells, use weights that are 2-1/2 to 5 pounds each. You will need two of each weight. Dumbbells can be purchased in any sporting goods store, and in most discount stores, such as Target or Wal-Mart.

(As you progress, you may find that you will need 8 to 10 pound dumbbells for some exercises.)

• Push ups
3 Sets   10-12 Reps

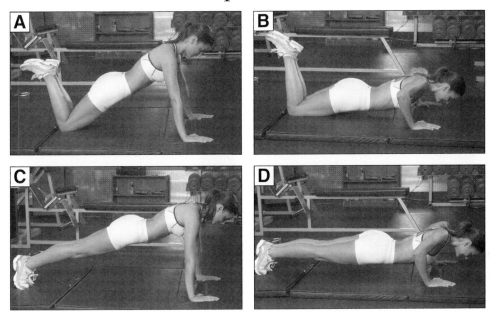

STEPS

1. Begin on your knees. Put your palms flat on the floor, arms shoulder-width apart, back flat. (A)

2. Lower yourself close to the floor, keeping your back as flat as possible. (B)

3. Push yourself back to the starting position. Repeat.

4. As you get stronger and can complete all reps from the knee position, transition to the more challenging foot position C and D.

KEEP IN MIND

• You may only be able to do a few at first. This is okay; you will improve quickly.

• Pullovers
3 Sets   10-12 Reps

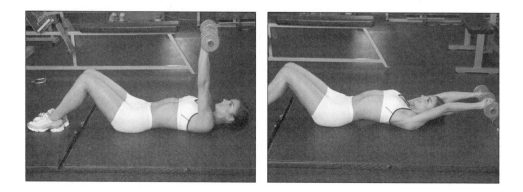

STEPS

1. Lie on your back with your knees bent, feet flat on the floor.

2. Holding the dumbbells with your palms facing toward your feet, extend your arms straight up (above your chest).

3. Keeping your arms as straight as possible, lower the dumbbells back, over your head to the floor (or as far as you can).

4. Raise back up to the starting position. Repeat.

KEEP IN MIND

• Stretch as far as possible, but do not stress your shoulders.

• Military press w/dumbbells
3 Sets   10-12 Reps

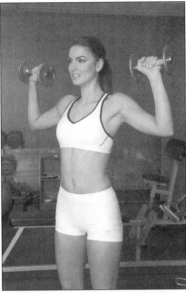

STEPS

1. Stand and hold your dumbbells at shoulder level, palms facing forward.

2. Press the weight up above your head until your arms are fully extended.

3. Lower the weight to the starting position, and repeat.

KEEP IN MIND

• Do your reps with very slow, very controlled movements to reduce the chance of injury.

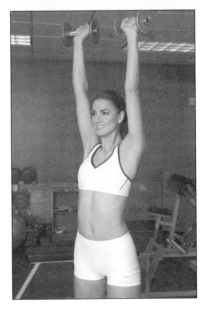

141

• Bicep curl
3 Sets   10-12 Reps

STEPS

1. Stand, and hold the dumbbells down by your sides with your palms facing forward.

2. Keeping your elbows positioned by your sides, raise the dumbbells up toward your shoulders as far as possible.

3. Slowly lower to the starting position, and repeat.

KEEP IN MIND

• Keep your elbows as your sides at all times during this exercise.

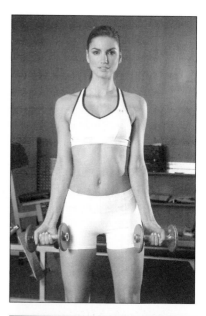

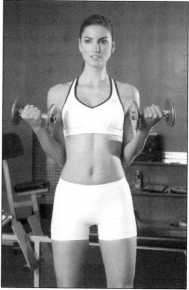

• Tricep kickback
3 Sets   10-12 Reps

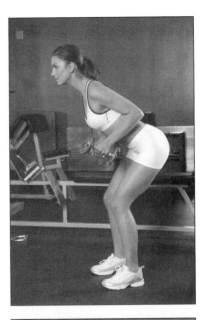

STEPS

1. From a standing position, bend over at the waist at a 45°-90° angle. Bend your knees slightly—this will eliminate lower back strain.

2. Keeping your elbows steady at your sides, push the dumbbells back until your arms are straight.

3. Lower slowly to the starting position, and repeat.

KEEP IN MIND

• Do not swing or move your elbows away from your side during this exercise.

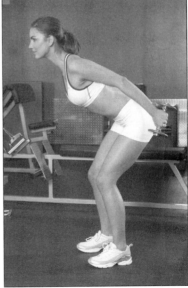

143

• Standing squats
3 Sets   10-12 Reps

STEPS

1. Stand with your feet shoulder width apart, hands by your sides.

2. Keeping your back straight and your chest out, lower yourself until your hips are at a 90° angle with your knees. (Your butt will push backward, and the final position is as if you are sitting in an imaginary chair.)

3. Push back up to the starting position, and repeat.

KEEP IN MIND

• Keep your back flat, not rounded forward.

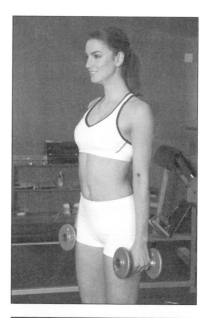

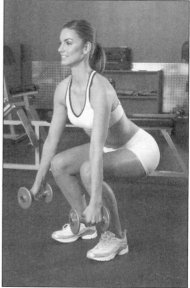

144

• Stationary lunges
3 Sets   10-12 Reps

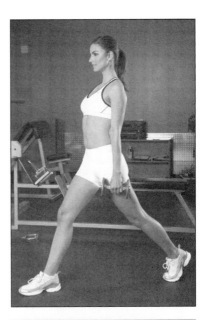

STEPS

1. Stand and hold the dumbbells by your sides.

2. Take a long stride forward with your right leg, and lower your rear left knee until it is just off the floor.

3. Push yourself back up to your original position.

4. Do 10 repetitions using the right leg, then 10 repetitions with the left leg.

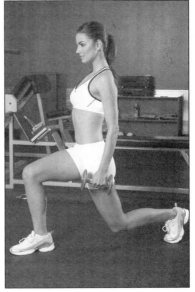

KEEP IN MIND

• For the first few days, start with no weight in your hands.

145

- ## Toe raises
  ## 3 Sets   10-12 Reps

STEPS

1. Stand with your dumbbells at your side.

2. Lift your heels until you are on the tip of your toes.

3. Lower back down to the floor. Repeat.

KEEP IN MIND

- Pause at the top of this movement to flex your calf muscles.

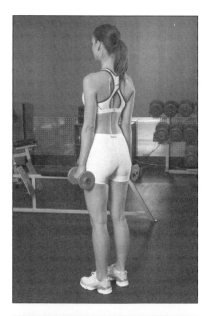

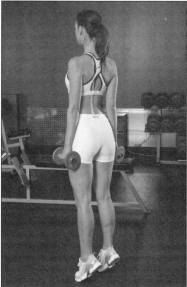

• Crunches
3 Sets   10-12 Reps

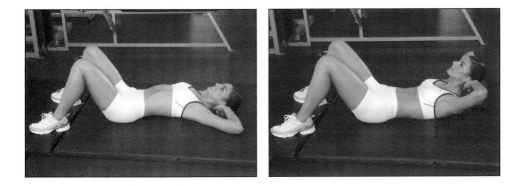

STEPS

1. Lie on your back with your knees bent and your feet on the floor. Place your hands behind your head or across your chest.

2. Lift your torso towards the ceiling. Breathe out on the upward movement.

3. Lower your torso and repeat.

KEEP IN MIND

• You should feel constant tension in your abs, not your neck or back.

Phase Two: Transition

**For HOME workout, do ALL exercises listed
for Phase One, PLUS one or two additional
exercises per muscle group. Do the exercises in
the order listed. (Photographs and descriptions
are only provided for the exercises that are
new additions to this phase.)**

- ## Push ups *(Home - Phase One)*
  ## 3 Sets   10-12 Reps

- ## Dumbbell flies
  ## 2 Sets   10-12 Reps

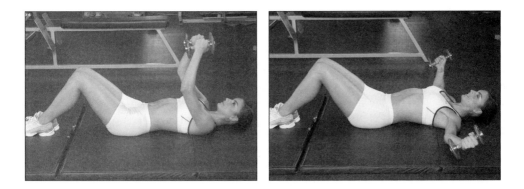

STEPS

1. Holding a dumbbell in each hand, lie on your back. Place your arms in a rounded position, with palms facing each other.

2. Lower your arms out to your sides, all the way to the floor.

3. Keeping your arms in the rounded position, return to the starting position. Repeat.

KEEP IN MIND

- While lowering the dumbbells to the floor, make sure to inhale and expand your ribcage.

- ## Pullovers *(Home - Phase One)*
  ## 3 Sets   10-12 Reps

- ## Single arm bent over row
  ## 2 Sets   10-12 Reps

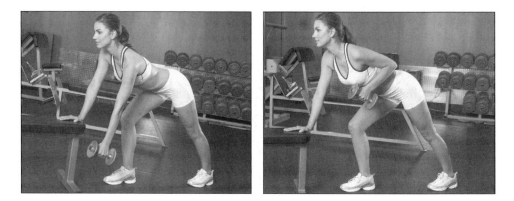

STEPS

1. From a standing position, step forward with your right leg. Bend at the waist until your body is parallel to the floor. Fully extend both arms straight down.

2. With your left arm, pull the dumbbell up to your side as if starting a lawnmower.

3. Lower to the starting position and repeat for all reps.

4. Return to a standing position. Step forward with your left leg, bend, extend your arms, and repeat the set using your right arm.

KEEP IN MIND

- Keep your back flat, not rounded. You should not feel stress on your lower back.

- **Military press w/dumbbells** *(Home - Phase One)*
  3 Sets   10-12 Reps

- **Side laterals**
  2 Sets   10-12 Reps

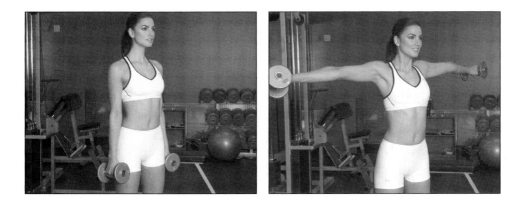

STEPS

1. Stand, holding the dumbbells at your sides with your palms facing inward.

2. Raise your arms out to your sides, lifting to a parallel position with your shoulders.

3. Lower the weight slowly to the starting position. Repeat.

KEEP IN MIND

- There should be a slight bend in your elbows. Only raise the dumbbells to a parallel position.

- **Bicep curl** *(Home - Phase One)*
  ## 3 Sets   10-12 Reps

- **Hammer curl**
  ## 2 Sets   10-12 Reps

STEPS

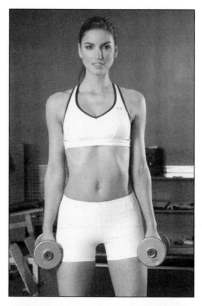

1. Stand and hold the dumbbells by your sides with your palms facing inward.

2. Keeping your elbows positioned by your sides, raise the dumbbells up as far as possible toward your shoulders.

3. Slowly lower the dumbbells to the starting position, and repeat.

KEEP IN MIND

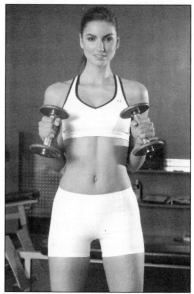

- Your hand position is very important on this exercise. Keep palms in to maintain the intensity on the right muscles.

- **Tricep kickback** *(Home - Phase One)*
  3 Sets   10-12 Reps

- **Single arm overhead extension**
  2 Sets   10-12 Reps

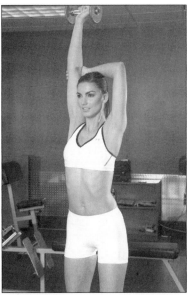

STEPS

1. From a standing position, hold a dumb bell in your right hand and extend your arm straight above your head.

2. Bending at the elbow, lower the dumb bell behind your head.

3. Return to the starting position, and repeat for all reps.

4. Repeat again, this time using your left arm.

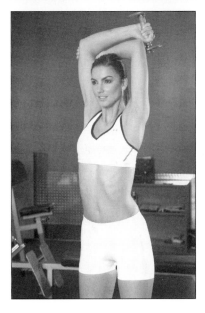

KEEP IN MIND

- Be careful not to hit your head.

- If this exercise is done properly, you should not feel stress in your shoulder.

153

- ## Standing squats *(Home - Phase One)*
  ### 2 Sets   10-12 Reps

- ## Stationary lunges
  (Home - Phase One)
  ### 2 Sets   10-12 Reps

- ## Walking lunges
  ### 2 Sets   10-12 Reps

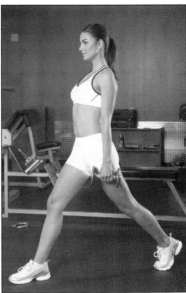

STEPS

1. Stand and hold the dumbbells by your sides.

2. Take a long stride forward and lower your rear knee until it is just off the floor.

3. Push yourself up, step forward with the other leg, and repeat the movement. Each step is counted as a repetition.

KEEP IN MIND

- For the first few times, start with no weight in your hands.

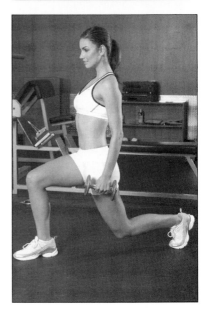

- ## Toe raises *(Home - Phase One)*
  ## 4 Sets   15 Reps

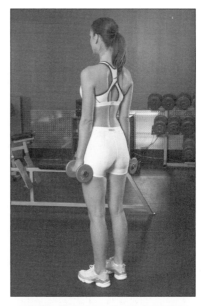

*Note: For Phase Two you will be doing
4 sets of this exercise instead of 3.*

STEPS

1. Stand with your dumbbells at
   your side.

2. Lift your heels until you are on the
   tip of your toes.

3. Lower back down to the floor.
   Repeat.

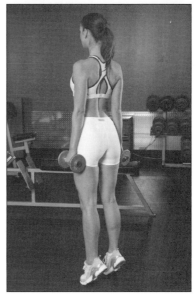

KEEP IN MIND

- Pause at the top of this movement
  to flex your calf muscles.

155

- ## Crunches *(Home - Phase One)*
  ## 3 Sets   10-12 Reps

- ## Leg lifts
  ## 3 Sets   10-12 Reps

STEPS

1. Lie on your back and place your arms down at your sides with your palms down.

2. Lift your legs 6 inches off of the ground, then bend your knees and pull your legs inward towards your chest. (Breathe out when you are pulling your legs inward.)

3. Extend your legs back out to the starting position, and repeat.

KEEP IN MIND

- You should only feel stress on your abdominals, not your neck or back.

157

Home

Phase Three: Energizing

For HOME workout, do ALL exercises listed for Phase One and Phase Two, PLUS one or two additional exercises per muscle group. Do the exercises in the order listed. (Photographs and descriptions are only provided for the exercises that are new additions to this phase.)

- ## Push ups *(Home - Phase One)*
  ### 2 Sets   10-12 Reps

- ## Dumbbell flies *(Home - Phase Two)*
  ### 2 Sets   10-12 Reps

- ## Dumbbell press
  ### 2 Sets   10-12 Reps

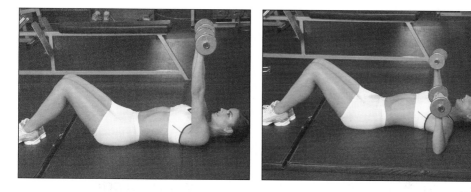

STEPS

1. Lie on your back on the floor.

2. Start with a dumbbell in each hand, palms facing your feet, and your arms straight and extended straight up over your chest.

3. Lower your elbows until they touch the ground.

4. Push back up to the starting position, and repeat.

KEEP IN MIND

- Inhale and expand your ribcage while lowering the dumbbells.

- Pullovers *(Home - Phase One)*
  2 Sets   10-12 Reps

- Single arm bent
  over row *(Home - Phase Two)*
  2 Sets   10-12 Reps

- Bent over
  underhand row
  2 Sets   10-12 Reps

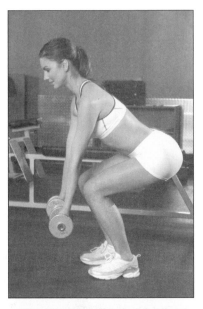

STEPS

1. From a standing position, bend
   over at the waist at a 45°-90° angle.
   Keep your knees slightly bent to
   alleviate stress in your lower back.

2. Holding a dumbbell in each hand,
   with your palms facing away from
   your body, extend your arms down
   toward the floor.

3. Pull both dumbbells up toward
   your waist at the same time.

4. Return to the starting position,
   and repeat.

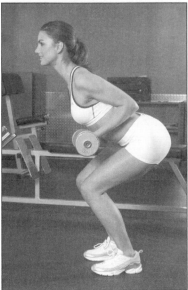

KEEP IN MIND

- Keep your back flat, not rounded.

- Military press w/dumbbells *(Home - Phase One)*
  2 Sets   10-12 Reps

- Side laterals *(Home - Phase Two)*
  2 Sets   10-12 Reps

- Rear delt raise
  2 Sets   10-12 Reps

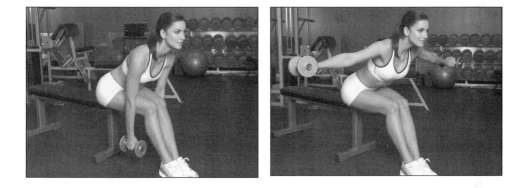

STEPS

1. Sit on the end of a chair or bench, and bend your torso over your knees. Hold the dumbbells with your palms facing inward.

2. Start with the dumbbells under your knees, and then raise them out to your sides. It is important to stay bent over.

3. Lower the dumbbells slowly to the starting position. Repeat.

KEEP IN MIND

- The stress is on your rear delts, not on your lower back.

161

- ## Bicep curl *(Home - Phase One)*
  ## 2 Sets   10-12 Reps

- ## Hammer curl
  (Home - Phase Two)
  ## 2 Sets   10-12 Reps

- ## Concentration curl
  ## 2 Sets   10-12 Reps

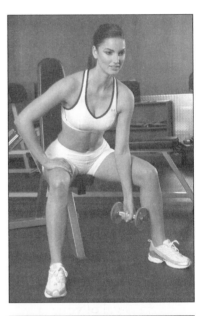

STEPS

1. Sit on the end of a chair or bench, with your feet spread apart.

2. Holding a dumbbell in your right hand, place your right elbow on the inside of your right thigh. (Your palm should face away from your body.)

3. Raise the dumbbell toward your shoulder, and squeeze your bicep at the top.

4. Lower the dumbbell slowly to the starting position. Repeat for all reps.

5. Then, repeat using your left arm.

KEEP IN MIND

- Keep your back flat, not rounded.

- Squeeze your bicep for a full second at the top.

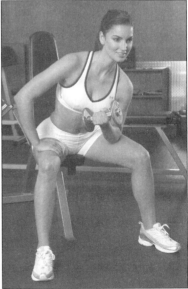

162

The Venus Summer Shape Up

- **Tricep kickback** *(Home - Phase One)*
  ## 2 Sets   10-12 Reps

- ## Single arm overhead extension
  (Home - Phase Two)
  ## 2 Sets   10-12 Reps

- ## Close grip wall press
  ## 2 Sets   10-12 Reps

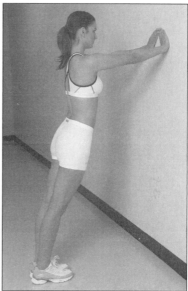

STEPS

1. Stand 20 to 30 inches from a wall. Place the palms of your hands close together against the wall at the level of your head.

2. Bend at the elbows and lower your face and torso toward the wall, like a standing push-up.

3. Before touching the wall with your face, push away until your elbows are fully extended, and then repeat.

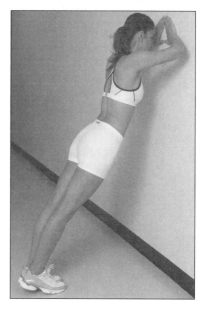

KEEP IN MIND

- For correct hand placement, spread your thumb away from your palm, then arrange your hands so that the tips of your thumbs touch each other, and the tips of your index fingers also touch each other— a triangle position.

163

- **Standing squats** *(Home - Phase One)*
  2 Sets   10-12 Reps

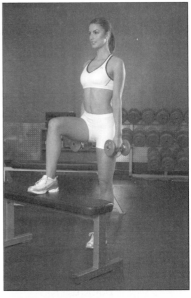

- **Stationary lunges**

  (Home - Phase One)
  2 Sets   10-12 Reps

- **Walking lunges**

  (Home - Phase Two)
  2 Sets   10-12 Reps

- **Step-ups on box OR**
  Plié squats
  2 Sets   10-12 Reps

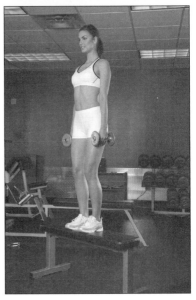

STEPS

Prep: You will need a box, step, or chair that is at least 15"-18" in height.

1. Step up with your right leg first, and follow with your left.

2. Then, step down with your left leg first.

3. Repeat until all 10-12 reps are complete on your right leg. Then repeat your 10-12 reps, leading with your left leg.

- ## Plié squats
  ## 2 Sets   10-12 Reps

STEPS

1. Stand with your feet very wide apart, with your toes pointing outward.

2. Hold a single dumbbell with both hands, and extend your arms straight down toward the floor.

3. Bend at the knees, and squat down until your hips are even with your knees.

4. Push back up to the starting position, and repeat.

KEEP IN MIND

- Your back should be flat, not rounded.

- Squeeze your glutes at the top of the movement for a full two seconds.

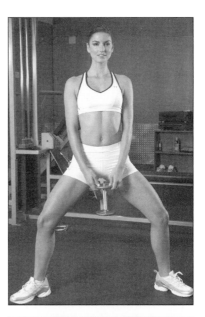

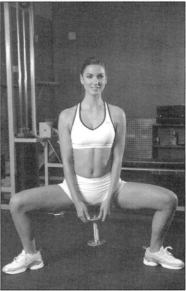

• Toe raises
4 Sets   25 Reps

STEPS

1. Stand with your dumbbells at your side.

2. Lift your heels until you are on the tip of your toes.

3. Lower back down to the floor. Repeat.

KEEP IN MIND

• Pause at the top of this movement to flex your calf muscles.

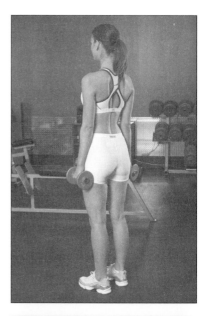

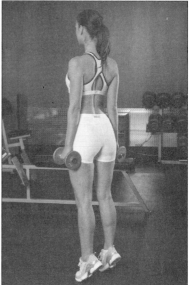

- ## Crunches *(Home - Phase One)*
  ## 2 Sets   10-12 Reps

- ## Leg lifts *(Home - Phase Two)*
  ## 2 Sets   10-12 Reps

- ## Core ball leg lift and Crunch
  ## 2 Sets   10-20 Reps

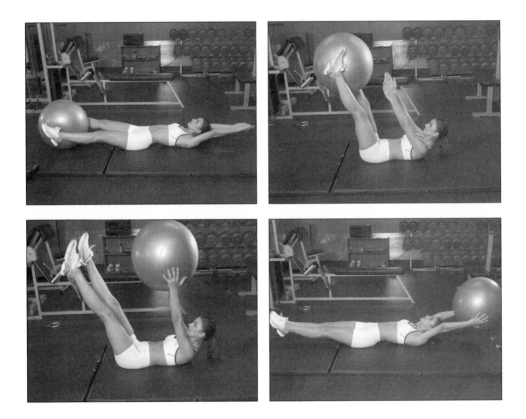

STEPS

1. Lie on your back with the core ball between your knees and ankles.

2. Lift your legs and torso simultaneously, and grab the ball with your hands.

3. Lower your torso and legs to the starting position, with the ball over your head.

4. Raise your torso and legs back up, and place the ball back between your knees and ankles.

5. Return to the starting position, and repeat.

KEEP IN MIND

• This is an advanced exercise--do your repetitions slowly and with great control.

Swiss Ball Exercises
for Super-Advanced
——————— ONLY!!! ———————

These exercises are quite difficult, and should only be performed if you have mastered the advanced levels of either the GYM or HOME exercise programs. You can purchase a Swiss Ball in the sports department of any discount department store, including Target and Wal-Mart.

The reason these exercises are difficult is because they require you to "balance" while performing the exercise. When you add the need to balance, you call upon your core muscles, so more muscles are working than when you do these same exercises on a rigid surface. To remain balanced, your form must be spot-on smooth, stable, and consistent.

If you wish to incorporate these exercises into your routine, REPLACE the exercise from the Gym or Home Phase Three with the comparable exercise from this section.

- ## Dumbbell Flies
  ## 3 Sets   10-12 Reps

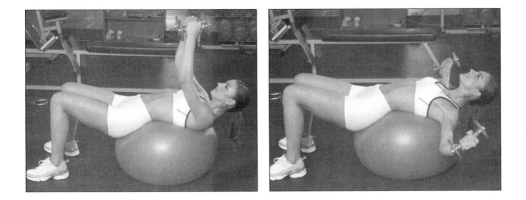

STEPS

1. Lie back over the ball. Position the ball in the middle of your back while planting your feet securely on the floor.

2. Hold a dumbbell in each hand, and place your arms in a rounded position.

3. Lower your arms out to your sides, keeping your arms in the rounded position.

4. Return to the starting position, and repeat.

KEEP IN MIND

- Do your repetitions slowly and in a very controlled manner.

• Dumbbell press
3 Sets   10-12 Reps

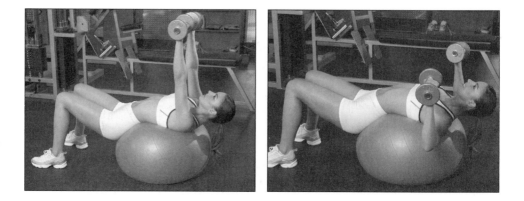

STEPS

1. Lie back over the ball. Position the ball in the middle of your back while planting your feet securely on the floor.

2. Start with a dumbbell in each hand, palms facing your feet, and your arms extended directly above your chest.

3. Lower the dumbbells until they are parallel with your chest.

4. Push back up to the starting position, and repeat.

KEEP IN MIND

• By balancing yourself on the ball, your body recruits its stabilizing muscles.

- ## Dumbbell pullover
  ## 3 Sets   10-12 Reps

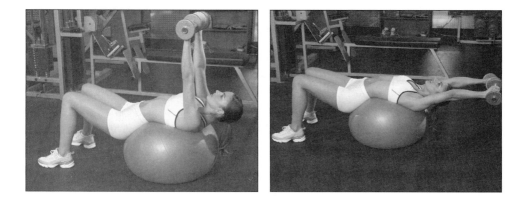

STEPS

1. Lie back over the ball.

2. Holding the dumbbells with your palms facing toward your feet, extend your arms straight up (above your chest).

3. Keeping your arms as straight as possible, lower the dumbbells back, over your head to the floor (or as far as you can).

4. Raise back up to the starting position. Repeat.

KEEP IN MIND

- Stretch as far as possible, but do not stress your shoulders.

173

• Military press
3 Sets   10-12 Reps

STEPS

1. Sit on the ball and plant your feet securely on the floor.

2. Hold the dumbbells at shoulder level, palms facing forward.

3. Press the weight up above your head until your arms are fully extended.

4. Lower the weight to the starting position, and repeat.

KEEP IN MIND

• Do your reps slowly to help you maintain your balance.

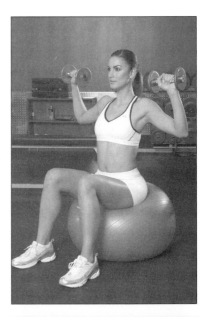

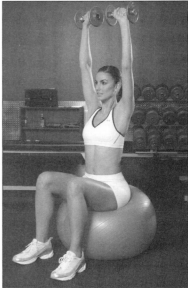

- ## Side laterals
  ## 3 Sets   10-12 Reps

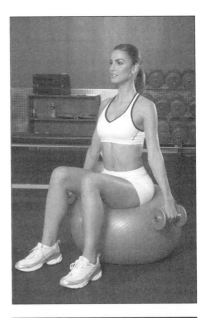

STEPS

1. Sit on the ball and plant your feet securely on the floor.

2. Hold your dumbbells at your sides with your palms facing inward.

3. Raise your arms out to your sides, until they are parallel with your shoulders.

4. Lower the weight slowly to the starting position, and repeat.

KEEP IN MIND

- There should be a slight bend in your elbows. Only raise the dumb-bells to a parallel position.

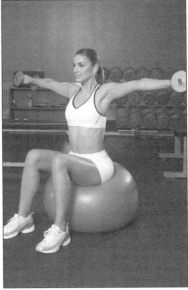

175

Exercise Summaries

Gym Workout, Phase One

Chest
Medium-grip barbell bench press
(page 103)

Back
Wide-grip front pull-down
(page 104)

Shoulders
Military press (page 105)

Biceps
Close-grip easy curl bar (page 106)

Triceps
Tricep press down overhand
(page 107)

Legs
Lying hamstring curl (page 108)
Thigh extension (page 109)

Calves
Standing calf machine (page 110)

Abs
Crunches (page 111)

Gym Workout, Phase Two

Chest

Medium-grip barbell bench press
(page 103)

Inner-pec press (page 113)

Back

Wide-grip front pull-down
(page 104)

Narrow-grip seated row (page 114)

Shoulders

Military press (page 105)

Side laterals (page 115)

Biceps

Close-grip easy curl bar (page 106)

Hammer curl (page 116)

Triceps

Tricep press down overhand
(page 107)

Tricep press down underhand
(page 117)

Legs

Lying hamstring curl (page 108)

Thigh extension (page 109)

Squat (page 118) OR Leg Press
(page 119)

Walking lunges (page 120)

Calves

Standing calf machine (page 121)

Abs

Crunches (page 111)

Leg lifts (page 122)

Gym Workout, Phase Three

Chest
Medium-grip barbell bench press
(page 103)
Inner-pec press (page 113)
Palms-in dumbbell press (page 125)

Back
Wide-grip front pull-down
(page 104)
Narrow-grip seated row (page 114)
Underhand grip pulldown
(page 126) OR assisted pull-up
(page 127)

Shoulders
Military press (page 105)
Side laterals (page 115)
Rear delt raise (page 128)

Biceps
Close-grip easy curl bar (page 106)
Hammer curl (page 116)
Cable curls (page 129)

Triceps
Tricep press down overhand
(page 107)
Tricep press down underhand
(page 117)
Easy curl bar extension lying down
(page 130)

Legs
Lying hamstring curl (page 108)
Thigh extension (page 109)
Squat (page 118) OR Leg Press
(page 119)
Walking lunges (page 120)
Straight leg dead lifts (page 132)
OR Step ups on box (page 133)

Calves
Standing calf machine (page 121)
Toe raises (page 134)

Abs
Crunches (page 111)
Leg lifts (page 122)
Core ball leg lift and Crunch
(page 136)

Home Workout, Phase One

Chest
Push ups (page 139)

Back
Pullovers (page 140)

Shoulders
Military press w/dumbbells
(page 141)

Biceps
Bicep curl (page 142)

Triceps
Tricep kickback (page 143)

Legs
Standing squats (page 144)
Stationary lunges (page 145)

Calves
Toe raises (page 146)

Abs
Crunches (page 147)

Home Workout, Phase Two

Chest

Push ups (page 139)

Dumbbell flies (page 149)

Back

Pullovers (page 140)

Single arm bent over row
(page 150)

Shoulders

Military press w/dumbbells
(page 141)

Side laterals (page 151)

Biceps

Bicep curl (page 142)

Hammer curl (page 152)

Triceps

Tricep kickback (page 143)

Single arm overhead extension
(page 153)

Legs

Standing squats (page 144)

Stationary lunges (page 145)

Walking lunges (page 154)

Calves

Toe raises (page 146)

Abs

Crunches (page 147)

Leg lifts (page 156)

The Venus Summer Shape Up

Home Workout, Phase Three

Chest
Push ups (page 139)
Dumbbell flies (page 149)
Dumbbell press (page 159)

Back
Pullovers (page 140)
Single arm bent over row
(page 150)
Bent over underhand row
(page 160)

Shoulders
Military press w/dumbbells
(page 141)
Side laterals (page 151)
Rear delt raise (page 161)

Biceps
Bicep curl (page 142)
Hammer curl (page 152)
Concentration curl (page 162)

Triceps
Tricep kickback (page 143)
Single arm overhead extension
(page 153)
Close grip wall press (page 163)

Legs
Standing squats (page 144)
Stationary lunges (page 145)
Walking lunges (page 154)
Step ups (page 164) OR
Plié squats (page 165)

Calves
Toe raises (page 166)

Abs
Crunches (page 147)
Leg lifts (page 156)
Core ball leg lift and Crunch
(page 168)

Super-Advanced ONLY!

Swiss Ball Exercises

Dumbbell flies (page 171)

Dumbbell press (page 172)

Dumbbell pullover (page 173)

Military press (page 174)

Side laterals (page 175)

Chapter 10:
A Model Story—Jessiqa

Jessiqa has a passion for art. Growing up in front of the camera, she developed an eye for framing the world in a way that reveals unusual beauty. In addition to modeling, Jessiqa is an accomplished photographer who specializes in cityscapes. Currently, she is studying film and is applying her skills to the acting world.

Modeling is in my blood. I started when I was only 8 years old, when I posed in local ads for departments stores like Macy's and Mervyn's. I didn't have that one "big break"; my career has been one of steady and consistent growth. I was in a Sunkist ad when I was 10, got my first cover for a German fashion magazine in my teens, and I have been in several TV commercials, including one for Dove soap. I've been modeling with *Venus* for seven years, which has been an amazing experience. *Venus* has given me the opportunity to go on photo shoots to some of the most beautiful places in the world, including Belize, Key West, the Dominican Republic, Islamorada and Vieques. I have been privileged to work with some of the best talent in the country, including *Venus* photographer Jorge Alvarez (who I think is a genius). Modeling has given me great opportunities to travel, meet interesting, talented people and see places that I never would have dreamed existed.

I think being a successful swimwear model takes hard work, good genes, and being in the right place at the right time. You have to be born with certain physical characteristics. I didn't choose to be 5'8" or have my particular facial features, but I'm certainly happy that it turned out that way. My height and facial features have propelled me into this career, but I have to stay active and eat right in order to keep my body in shape for the camera.

Balanced Eating

My parents and grandparents always ate healthfully, so I had their examples as a strong foundation. I love food, but I'm very conscious of what I put into my body. One of my favorite mantras is, "My body is a temple." I try to think about this and act accordingly. I don't have a particularly strict diet, but I try, whenever possible, to eat whole foods—fresh vegetables, fresh fruit, and whole wheat. I don't eat poultry, pork, or beef, so I get my protein from fish, legumes, eggs, cheese, nonfat milk, soymilk (I drink a lot of soymilk), and nuts. I do have a sweet tooth, especially for ice cream. I think it's very important to eat the things you like, but with the intention not to overindulge.

I don't have any special diet advice, but I do believe it's necessary to keep your metabolism going. I never starve myself. I let my body tell me when I need to eat. I usually eat several small meals throughout the day. In the morning I make my own breakfast concoction of nonfat plain yogurt, blueberries, raspberries, some muesli, almonds, banana, and (if I want something sweet) a little honey. If I'm going to have a big meal, I like to have it in the earlier part of the day. My usual dinner is a salad, lots of veggies, not too much bread. I never use salad dressings; they're too heavy and add unwanted and unneeded calories. My favorite carbs include couscous, whole wheat bread, tortillas, pita bread and rice. I also love all kinds of cheeses—Feta, Brie, Havarti—I'm always on the hunt for something new, beyond the usual Cheddar.

Another important note is to drink a lot of water. This keeps my system hydrated and helps curb my appetite when I know I am not really hungry. I also drink a lot of green tea. I like varying the foods I eat so I get everything I want and everything my body needs. I find that if I eat right and focus on eating the right foods (and avoiding the bad ones), I never have to feel hungry.

Staying active

I grew up playing soccer and softball. Activities keep me balanced, especially when things may not be going well. My sense of well-being, my spirit, my energy, and my thought processes all depend on how active I am. Still, I try not to push too hard—exercise is about feeling good, not about pain. Now, I also enjoy yoga, which is about elongating my muscles and opening my joints. It adds to my routine in a different way than any other exercise. Yoga is very demanding and forces me to focus my attention on the moment, my breath, and my body. With each breath I feel as if I am releasing stress and tension from my body and mind.

Being a model has given me great incentive to develop a lifestyle that keeps me in shape. However, I do believe I would continue to make the right choices to maintain good health and balance even if I were in a different career. I have many interests outside of modeling—photography, acting, painting, and film-making,—all requiring time and creative energy. I find that eating the right foods and exercising give me prolonged energy to do all the things I want to do in life. In many ways, taking care of your body is like creating a great piece of art. It takes time, effort, hard work and a strong goal. You don't have to be a model to want to treat your body as though it were priceless!

Jessiqa's model secrets...

- Believes in eating whole foods—fresh fruits and vegetables, whole grains, legumes.

- Doesn't eat meat.

- Favorite dinner is a big salad with lots of different vegetables, no salad dressing, and maybe a whole wheat tortilla or rice.

- Exercises every day.

- Main activities are running and yoga. Often runs for 1 hour during a workout.

- Likes to run outdoors, where she feels more connected with the world.

Chapter 11:
Measuring Success

If you have followed the *Venus* program for the full 60 days, then you absolutely know it works. I'm willing to bet that there is a noticeable difference in the way you see yourself in the mirror, in the way you carry yourself, and in the admiring comments of friends and family. How many times in the past week has someone said to you, "Wow, you look different"? That's a pretty good feeling, isn't it? We all have an ego, and it feels great for others to notice our efforts and our accomplishments. But even more important than that is for you to ask yourself this question:

How do YOU feel about YOURSELF?

Ultimately, to make any real lifelong change—to truly change yourself— you must do it for <u>you</u>. Doing something for others may work in the short term, but that seldom leads to true long-term change. You have to want something better for yourself, and I hope you now see it. Take some time to celebrate your accomplishment!

I'm hoping this physical transformation gives you the motivation to continue practicing the fitness lessons you've learned. While this is a 60-day program, the reality is that the swimsuit models who work for *Venus* for 10 to 12 years follow this type of program their whole lives. My hope is that you use this experience as a stepping stone for a true lifestyle change, one that will allow you to stay physically active and to eat with your head and not your heart.

Do you remember back when I asked you to write down your goal? You have taken the first steps to getting there. The results you see in the mirror are proof that you can do it. The fact that you finished the program is proof that you cherish yourself, your body, your health, and your future. Look what you have done in just 60 days—imagine what you could do in a year, or three years! And the best part is that the benefits are self-reinforcing. If you see results, you are more likely to have the will and the desire to keep doing what works. Results will make you stronger, and you won't understand how you ever could have doubted yourself.

You are on your way to the Beach!

But of course, there is more to your transformation than just the physical change, isn't there? This program has two main goals, but I've hidden one of them until now. The first is to help you become healthier and fitter. (That one is obvious.) The second goal is to help you release your personal potential.

If you are like most people, you probably felt "stuck" in a body you weren't happy with, "stuck" with a defeatist attitude, and "stuck" in your own personal rut. You probably had become resigned and thought there was nothing you could do improve yourself. Now you know—like I know—that it's just not true.

So much of life is all about attitude. If you tell yourself, "This is just the way I am, there's nothing I can do, I'm stuck," then guess what—you are absolutely right. It becomes a self-fulfilling prophecy. Attitude makes all the difference in life. It doesn't matter what your problems are—your attitude makes life either a bowl of cherries or a bowl of pits.

Life is about the attitude that we carry with us. When the circumstances we are fighting or facing are negative ones, a positive attitude is even more important. If you can turn the attitude around, then everything changes. Tasks are easier, anxiety and worry are weakened, and it is easier to remake yourself.

Most people aren't stuck physically; they are stuck mentally. They don't believe they can do anything to change their current circumstance. They become stuck on that one particular "branch of the tree" and don't realize that with a little bit of effort they can climb someplace else. But you know you can climb higher. You've done it! You completed a tough 60-day program. You've started to remake your body and your life. You know that anything is possible, and how high you climb is entirely up to you. That's the true measure of success. That's the *Venus* attitude.

The Venus Summer Shape Up

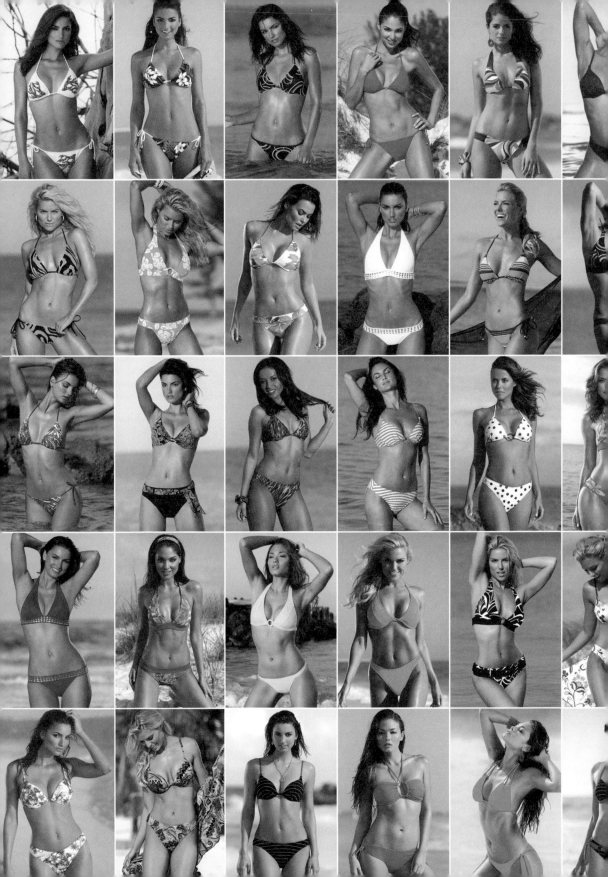

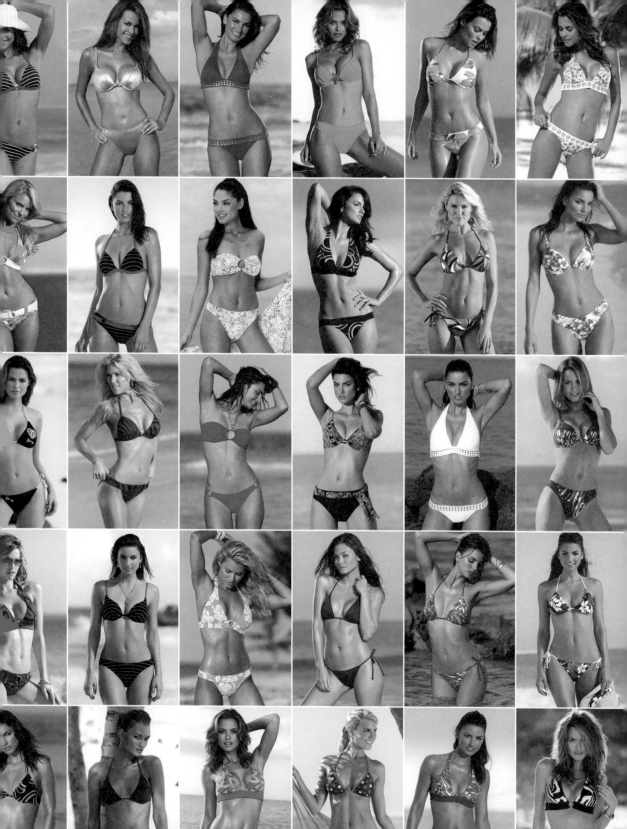